LOW FODMAP
SNACKS for
Irritable Bowel Syndrome

1

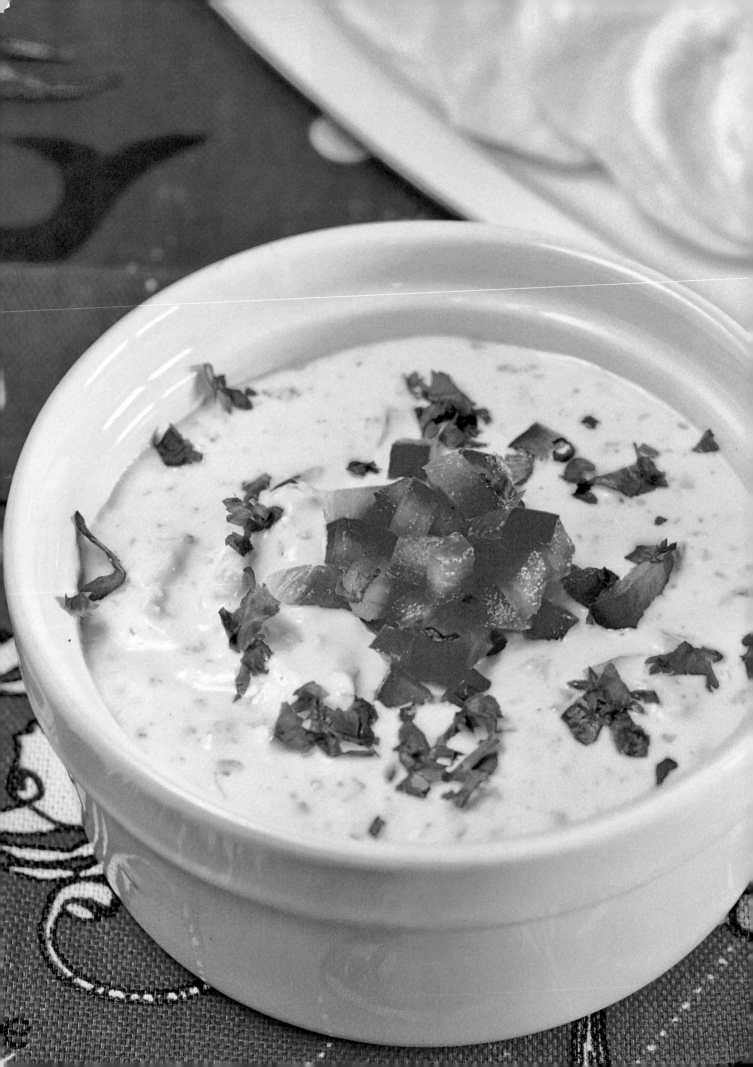

LOW FODMAP
SNACKS for
Frritable Bowel Syndrome

SUZANNE PERAZZINI

CREATOR OF *STRANDS OF MY LIFE*

photography & recipes by Suzanne Perazzini

LOW FODMAP
SNACKS for
Irritable Bowel Syndrome

Written by: Suzanne Perazzini
Produced by: Suzanne Perazzini

www.strandsofmylife.com
suzanne.perazzini@orcon.net.nz

© 2014

COPYRIGHT

Design, Art Direction, Edited and Produced by Suzanne Perazzini

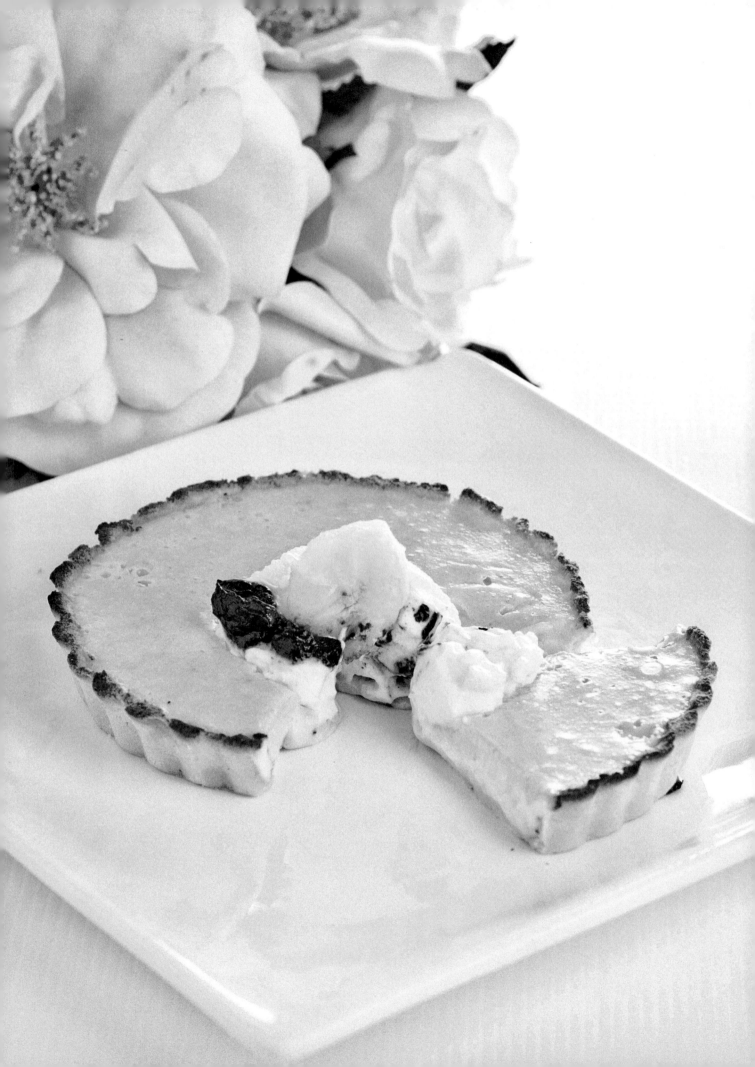

Contents

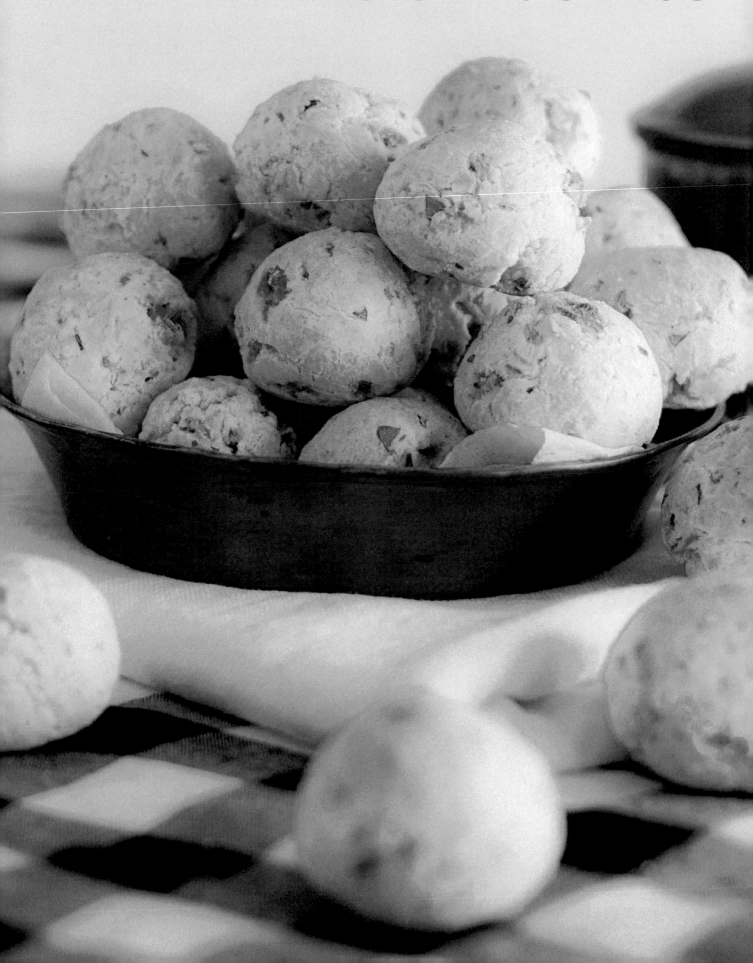

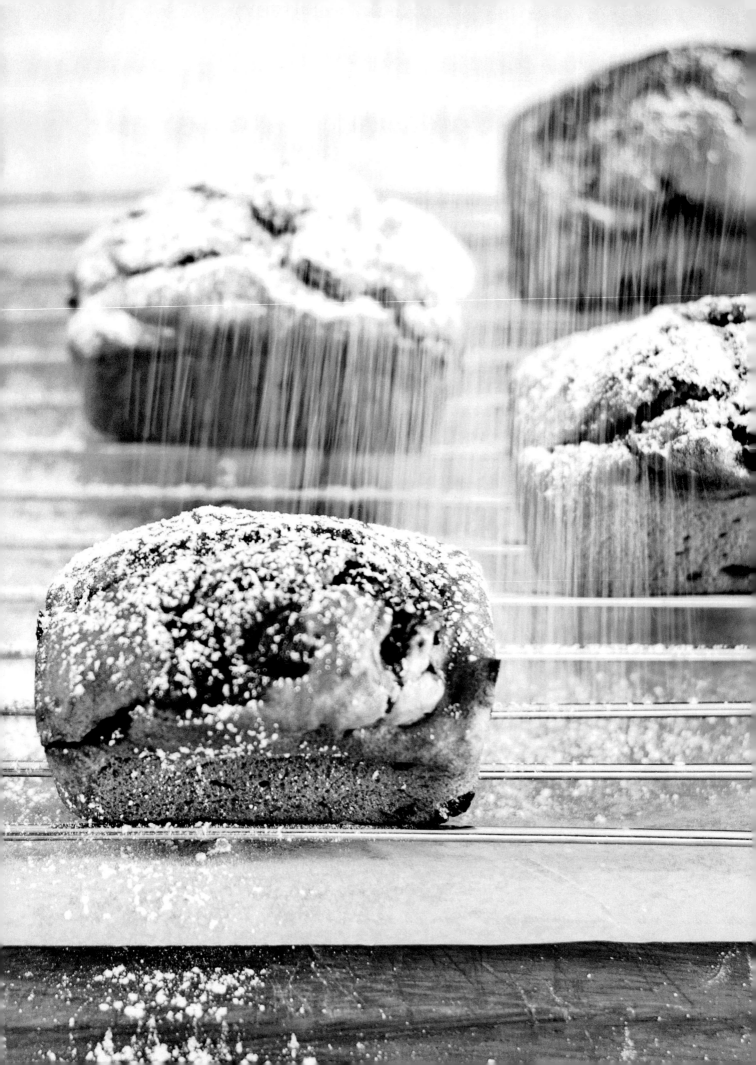

Introduction

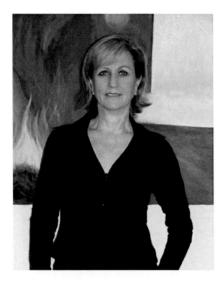

My name is Suzanne Perazzini and I am a super organized perfectionist who is a lover of travelling, reading, writing, photography and cooking. I live with my Italian husband and 24-year-old son in New Zealand in a house overlooking the Pacific Ocean.

I have suffered from digestive issues all my life. Through the years, I approached numerous doctors with my symptoms only to be told that I had irritable bowel syndrome and to eat more fibre, whole grains, fruit and vegetables. Each time I diligently went away and obeyed their instructions and felt worse than ever. They say that the definition of insanity is doing the same thing over and over and expecting a different result. I guess I was insane. For years!

A few years ago, I started my blog, Strands of My Life, as a way of exploring food and the effect it had on me. I tried various different diets and one day I Googled the heck out of my symptoms for the zillionth time, and the low FODMAP diet came onto my radar, and I realised I had seen it mentioned before but had glossed over it. I found an article that described the symptoms of someone who was intolerant to FODMAPs and I had a light bulb moment. This person was describing me, right down to how 'healthy' food made them worse. I investigated further and fructose malabsorption was mentioned. I knew almost immediately that I had hit the bullseye. The puzzle pieces were falling into place. I read about the hydrogen breath test for fructose malabsorption and had soon booked myself in for one. The test was positive. I was put onto a nutritionist who specialized in the low Fodmap diet, and I started the elimination portion of it. The improvement was rapid and surprising and miraculous. Some days I thought I could dance on water.

Almost two years later, there are days when I think I am feeling so good that I can test the limits of this diet, but then the symptoms return and I remember what it used to be like. I now blog, not to find a solution to my own issues, but so I can help others like me who are suffering and have suffered all their lives. This intolerance is a strange and difficult one to isolate. I had tried eliminating so many types of food in the past with no relief but I had never thought of something as complex as this. For the healthiest foods to be the culprits is almost unthinkable, and I now know why the doctors' advice always made me worse.

I have written this cookbook to help out those of you who, like me, must stick to the low FODMAP diet but struggle to come up with snack ideas.

I am the creator of the Inspired Life Low Fodmap Coaching Program to help those who are struggling with their IBS and the diet. If you would like to learn more about the program, have a look at this page: www.strandsofmylife.com/coachingprogram. You will find a link near the bottom which will take you to an application form. Once I have received the form, I will give you a call to discuss your individual situation.

I hope you enjoy making these recipes.

Best wishes,

Suzanne

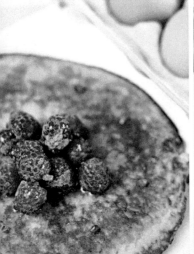
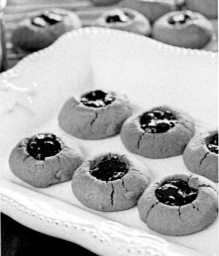
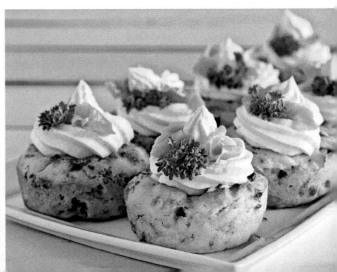

What are low FODMAPs?

FODMAP stands for Fermentable Oligo-saccharides, Disaccharides, Mono-saccharides and Polyols).

Fermentable:
The process through which gut bacteria break down undigested carbohydrate to produce gases (hydrogen, methane and carbon dioxide).

Oligo-saccharides:
Fructo-oligosaccarides (FOS) found in wheat, rye, onions and garlic.

Galacto-oligosaccharides (GOS):
Found in legumes/pulses.

Disaccharides:
Lactose found in milk, soft cheese, yoghurts etc.

Mono-saccharides:
Fructose (in excess of glucose) found in honey, many fruits and vegetables, high fructose corn syrups etc.

Polyols:
Sugar polyols (eg. sorbitol, mannitol) found in some fruit and vegetables and used as artificial sweeteners.

On the following pages you will find the foods (and amounts) you can eat on the low Fodmap diet. The research is ongoing and, with time, more foods will be added to the list of allowable foods.

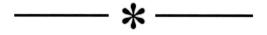

Vegetables

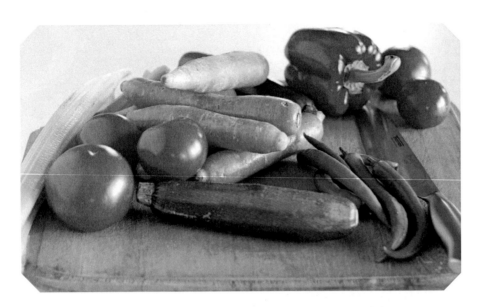

- alfalfa sprouts (½ cup)
- bean sprouts (½ cup)
- beetroot (2 slices)
- bok choy (1 cup)
- broccoli (½ cup)
- Brussel sprouts (2)
- cabbage-common (1 cup)
- cabbage-savoy (½ cup)
- bell peppers (½ cup)
- carrot (1)
- celeriac (½)
- celery (¼ stalk)
- chicory leaves (½ cup)

- red chilli (1)
- chives (1 tbsp)
- choy sum (1 cup)
- cucumber (½ cup)
- eggplant (½ cup)
- endive leaves (4)
- fennel leaves (½ cup)
- fennel bulb (½ cup)
- ginger root (1 tsp)
- green beans (10)
- kale (1 cup)
- leeks - green part (½ cup)
- lettuce (1 cup)

- okra (3 pods)
- peas (¼ cup)
- potato (1)
- pumpkin (½ cup)
- radishes (2)
- seaweed, Nori (2 sheets)
- silverbeet (1 cup)
- snow peas (5 pods)
  spinach (1 cup)
- spring onion - green part (1 bunch)
- squash (2)
- sweet potato (½ cup)
- tomato (1)
- turnips (1 cup)
- water chestnuts
1. (½ cup)
- witlof (4 leaves)
- zucchini (½ cup)

Fruits

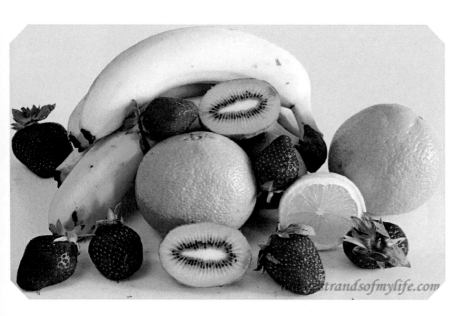

- honeydew (1/2 cup)
- kiwifruit (1)
- lemon juice (1 tsp)
- mandarins (2)
- oranges (1)
- passionfruit (1)
- paw paw (1/2 cup)
- pear, prickly (1)
- pineapple (1/2 cup)
- raspberries (10)
- rhubarb (1/2 stalk)
- strawberries (8)

- bananas (1)
- blueberries (20)
- cantaloup (1/2 cup)

- dragon fruit (1)
- durian (2 segments)
- grapes (20)

———— ————

Dried Fruit

- banana (10 chips)
- coconut milk (1/2 cup)

- shredded coconut (1/4 cup)

- cranberries (1 tbsp)
- pawpaw (1 piece)

13

Grain

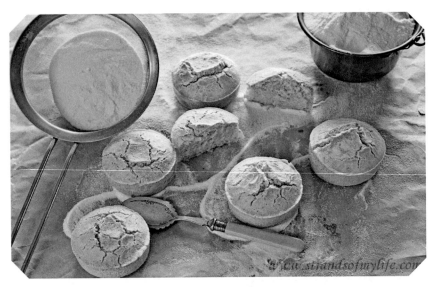

- gluten-free pasta (1 cup)
- polenta (1 cup)
- quinoa (1 cup)
- quinoa flakes (1 cup)
- white rice (1 cup)
- rice noodles (1 cup)
- sorghum
- sourdough oat bread (1 slice)
- puffed rice (1/2 cup)
- sourdough spelt bread (2 slices)

- gluten-free bread
- gluten-free cereals
- amaranth
- arrowroot
- brown rice (1 cup)
- buckwheat
- corn
- millet
- oats, dry (1/4 cup)
- oat bran (2 tbsp)

——— ✳ ———

Legumes/Pulses

- canned chickpeas (1/4 cup)
- canned lentils (1/2 cup)
- boiled lentils, green/red (1/4 cup)

Milk Products

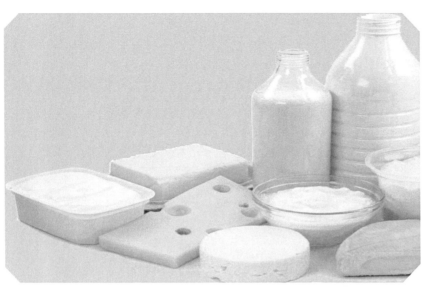

- feta (1/2 cup)
- haloumi (50gms/1.8oz)
- hard cheeses (40gms/1.4oz)
- lactose-free milk
- lactose-free yoghurt (1 small tub)
- ricotta (2 tbsp)
- soy milk, from soy bean protein (1 cup)
- cheddar (40gms/1.4oz)
- cottage cheese (4 tbsp)

Drinks

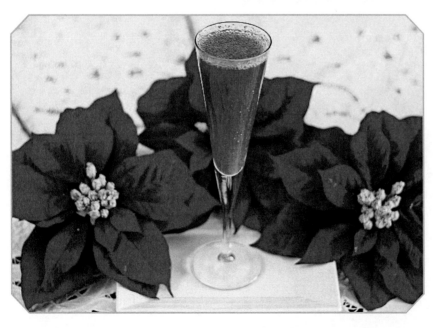

- orange juice (½ glass)
- red wine (1 glass)
- sparkling white wine (1 glass)
- vegetable - (1 glass)
- white wine, dry (1 glass)
- beer (1 can)
- cranberry juice (1 glass)

Sweeteners

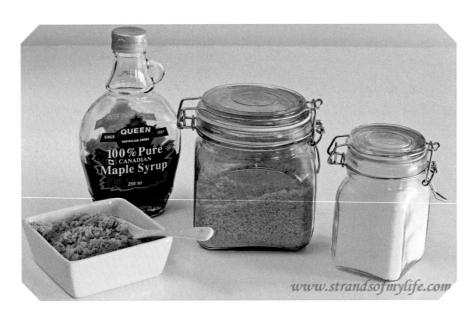

- maple syrup
- marmalade (2 tbsp)
- rice bran syrup
- stevia
- strawberry jam (2 tbsp)
- sugar (sucrose)

- artificial sweeteners not ending in -ol
- glucose
- golden syrup

———— ————

Protein Sources

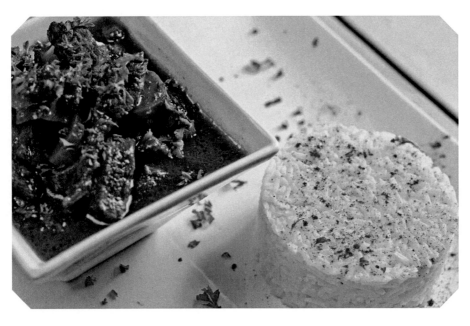

- chicken (125gms/4.4oz)
- eggs (2)
- fish (125gms/4.4oz)
- meat (125gms/4.4oz)
- tempeh (150gms/5.3oz)
- tofu - firm (1 cup)

Spices

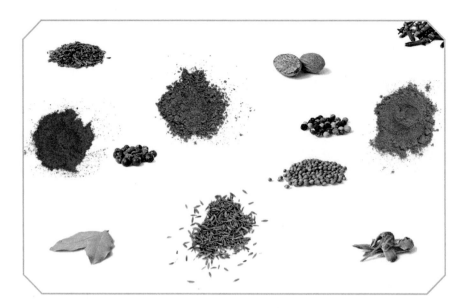

- cinnamon (1 tsp)
- coriander (1 tsp)
- cumin (1 tsp)
- five spice (1 tsp)
- turmeric (1 tsp)

———— ✳ ————

Sauces

- balsamic vinegar (1 tbsp)
- barbeque sauce (2 tbsp)
- fish sauce (1 tbsp)
- garlic-infused oil (2 tsp)
- mustard (1 tbsp)
- oyster sauce (1 tbsp)
- peanut butter (2 tbsp)
- soy sauce (2 tbsp)
- tahini paste (1 tbsp)
- vegemite (1 tsp)

———— ✳ ————

Herbs (1 cup)

- basil
- chives
- coriander
- parsley
- rosemary
- tarragon
- thyme

Advice for those eating a Low Fodmap diet

- Hunger is your enemy so eat five small meals a day which all include protein and fat (limited because fat is a gut irritant) to give you long-lasting energy.

- Keep low Fodmap snacks with you in case you get hungry and could be tempted by the wrong foods.

- Leave 3 to 5 hours between meals as this helps stimulate the migrating motor complex.

- Keep to a regular eating routine so your body learns what to expect.

- Eat only 2-3 pieces of low Fodmap fruit per day and space them out.

- Make sure you don't eat too many low Fodmap vegetables in one sitting. They could add up to a high Fodmap mix.

- Caffeine and alcohol are gut irritants and should be consumed in limited amounts.

- Carbonation is a gut irritant so avoid carbonated drinks.

- Keep up your water and fat intake to prevent constipation but don't overdo it as fat is a gut irritant.

- Proteins like meat, chicken and fish don't contain Fodmaps so you can increase the amounts you eat to keep away hunger.

- The best drink is water – it contains no Fodmaps.

- Avoid processed food because of the additives which could be gut irritants. If you don't recognize an ingredient as a food item, put the product back on the shelf.

- Take probiotics only if you are sure that you have low gut bacteria. If you have SIBO (small intestinal bacterial overgrowth), probiotics will make the situation worse.

- Make sure that you keep up your calcium intake through calcium-fortified dairy replacements and other calcium-rich foods.

- Make sure you don't eat while doing other activities. Take time out to eat in a peaceful environment so you are relaxed, which means your gut is relaxed.

- Stand up for yourself when someone urges you to eat a food which will hurt you. Tell them clearly that it will make you sick. Don't leave any room for doubt.

SAVOURY
SNACKS
— ✱ —

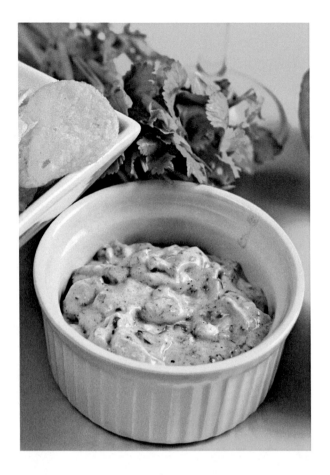 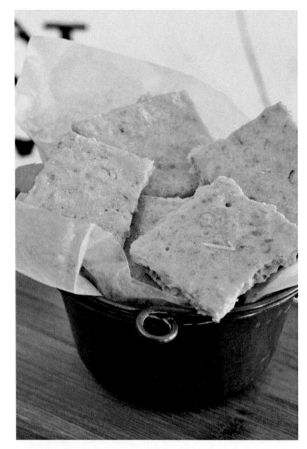

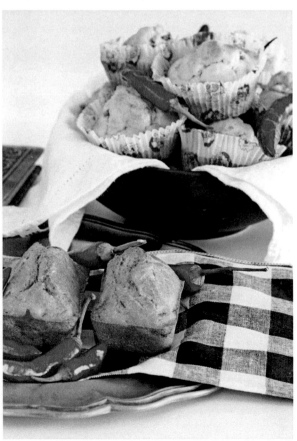 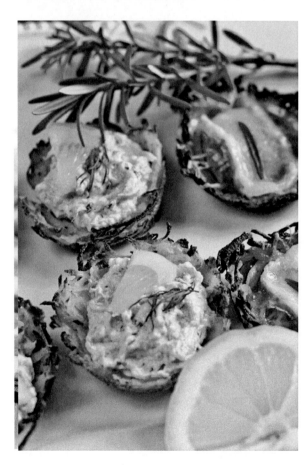

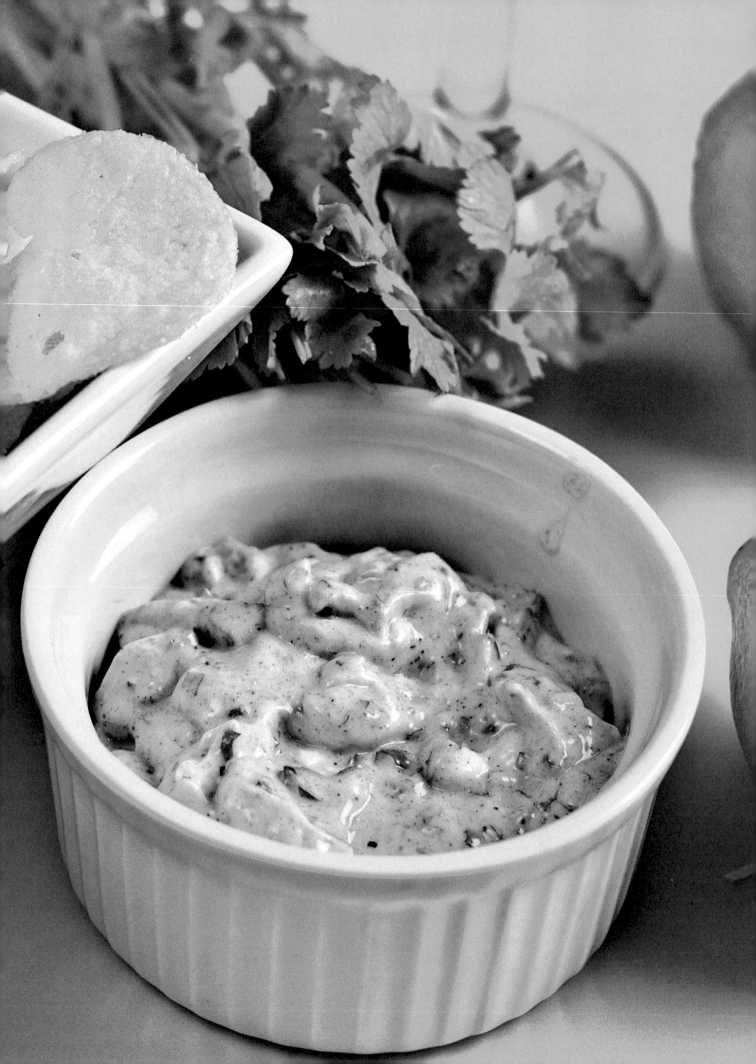

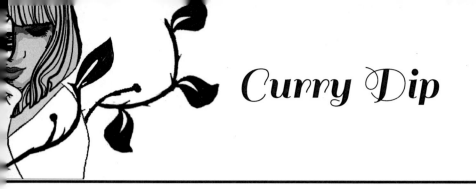

Curry Dip

Ingredients

¼ cup of lactose-free Greek yoghurt
½ cup mayonnaise
2 spring onions - green part only
1 tsp garam masala
1 tsp cumin powder
1 tsp coriander powder
1 tbsp oil
1 tbsp fresh coriander, chopped finely
6 drops of hot sauce
1 tsp lemon juice
Salt & pepper

Instructions

1. Heat the oil in a frying pan and add the spring onions chopped finely and the spices.
2. Cook for 1 minute.
3. Add all the ingredients together.
4. Serve with chips or fresh vegetable sticks.

Strands of My Life

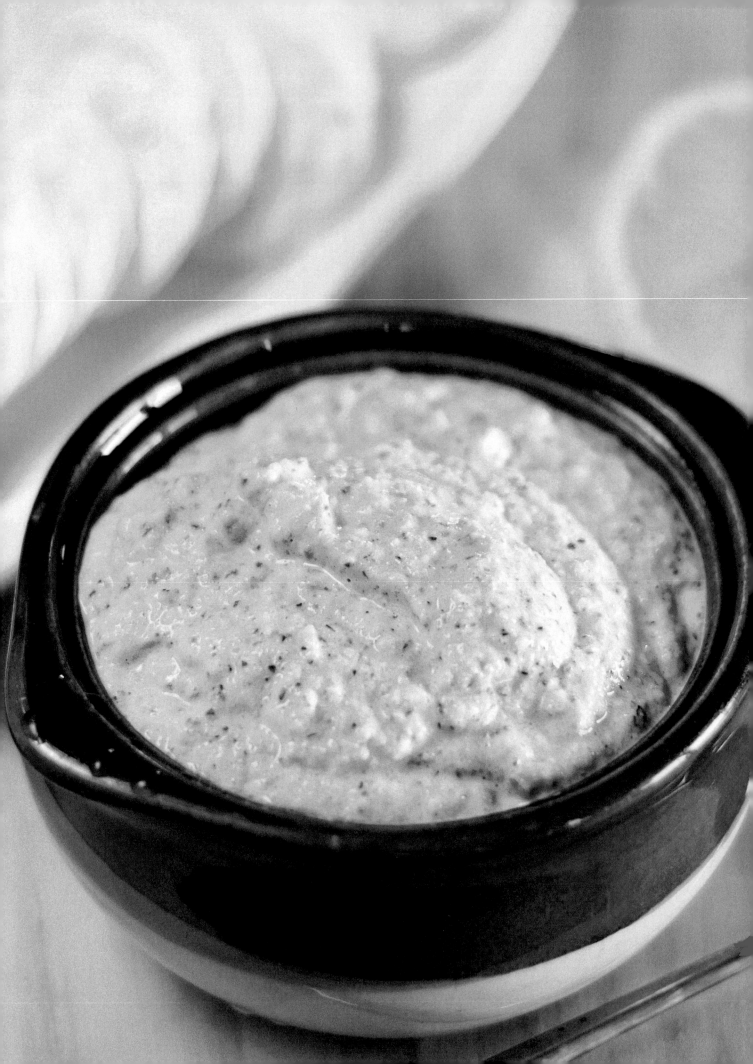

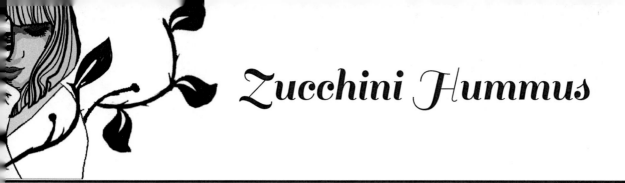

Zucchini Hummus

Ingredients

2 cups chopped zucchini
½ cup tahini
Juice of 2 lemons
1 tsp dried cumin
1 tsp turmeric
1 tsp dried coriander
1 tsp salt

Instructions

1. Process all the ingredients together in a food processor.
2. Serve with raw vegetable crudités or gluten-free crackers.
3. Keep in the fridge.

Strands of My Life

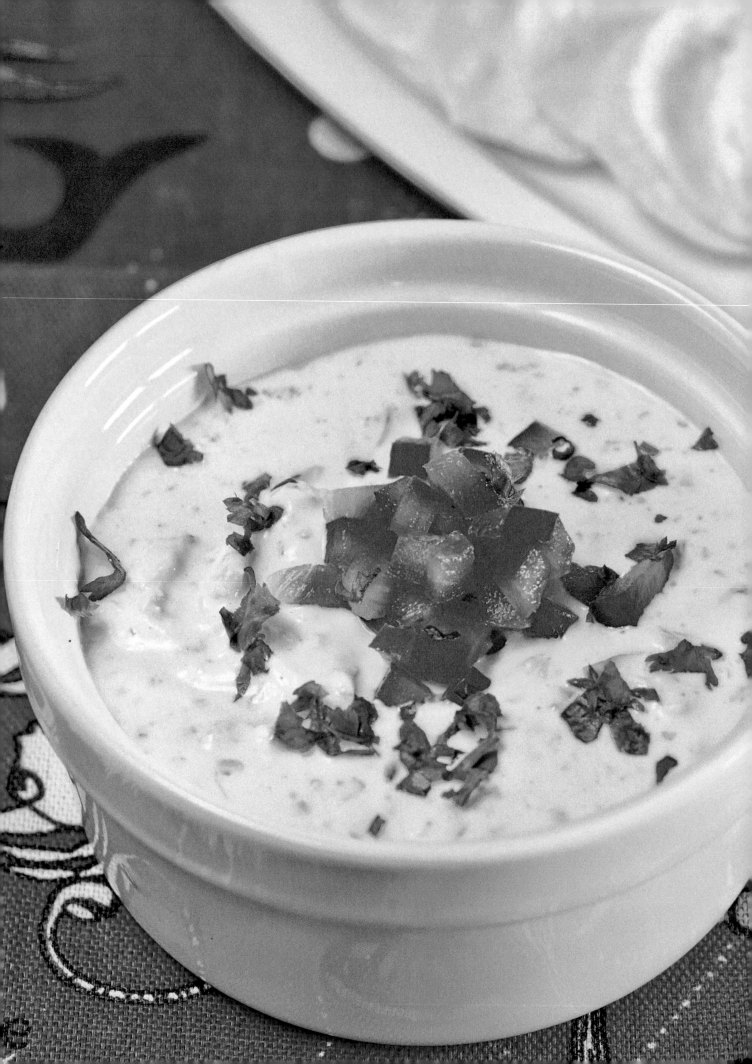

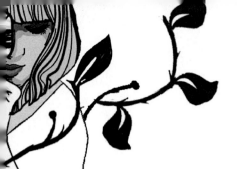

Feta & Bacon Dip

Ingredients

250gms/8.8oz feta cheese
½ red bell pepper
2 slices of thick bacon, grilled and chopped small
1 tbsp chopped coriander
Black pepper

Instructions

1. Place the feta, black pepper and coriander in a small processor and process until smooth.
2. Chop up the red pepper roughly and add to the processor.
3. Process a little to just chop up the red pepper.
4. Turn out into a serving bowl and add the bacon and fold in.
5. Keep in the fridge.

Note: 1/2 cup of feta is low Fodmap

Strands of My Life

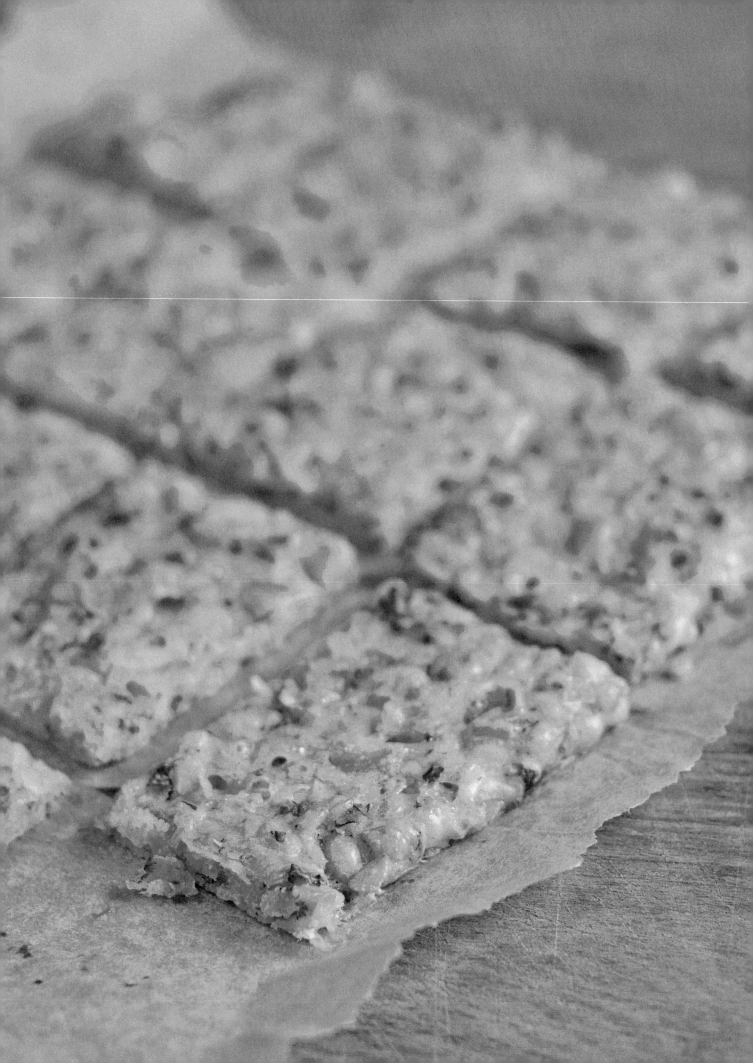

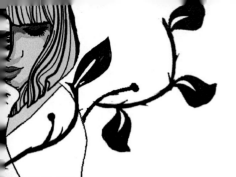

Camembert Parsley Crackers

Ingredients

1 cup rice flakes
1/2 cup chickpea flour (a small amount is low Fodmap)
1/2 tsp salt
2 tbsp fresh parsely, chopped finely
1/4 cup oil
2 eggs
80gms/3 oz Camembert cheese

Instructions

1. Heat oven to 180°C/350°F.
2. Combine the dry ingredients and the parsley in a bowl.
3. Chop up the cheese finely and add to the dry ingredients.
4. Beat the eggs and oil together.
5. Mix the wet and dry ingredients together.
6. Place a sheet of baking paper on an oven tray.
7. Spread the mixture out on the paper as thin as possible without creating holes. Shape it into a rectangle.
8. Place in the oven and cook for 10-15 minutes until golden and crisp.
9. Slice into square biscuits as soon as it is out of the oven and let them cool.
10. Eat fresh.

Note: The next day, freshen them up, by placing in a hot pan, and crisping up on both sides.

Makes 12 crackers

Strands of My Life

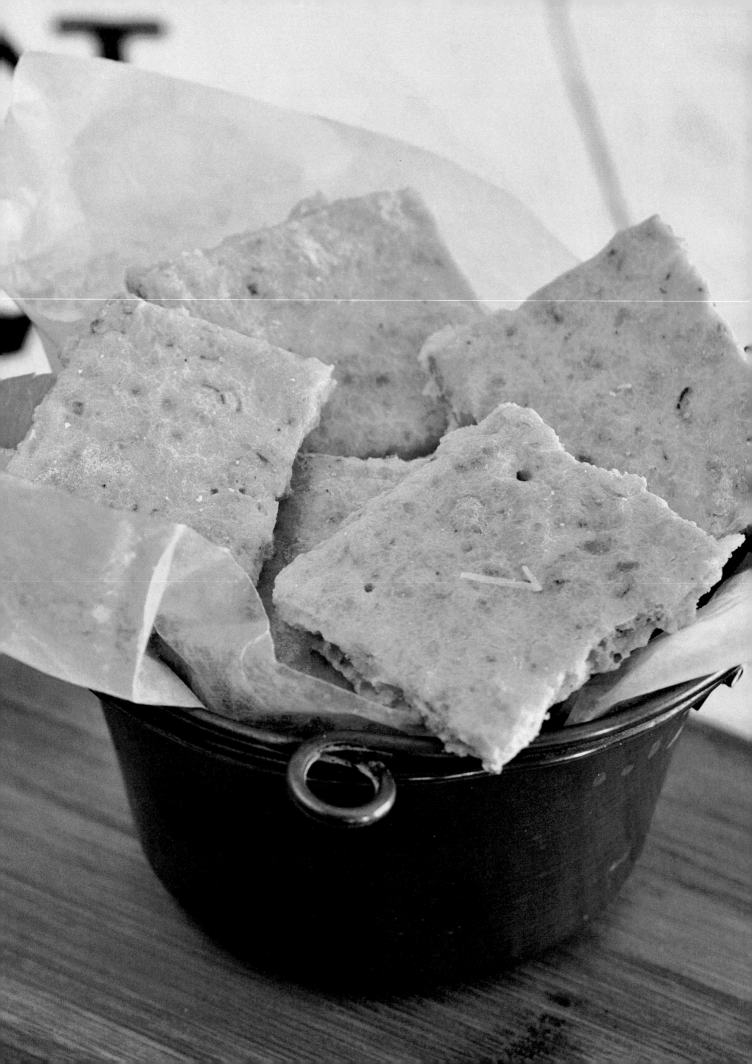

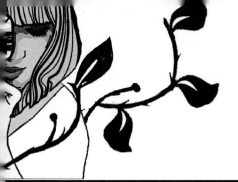

Parmesan Rice Flake Crackers

Ingredients

1 cup rice flakes
¼ cup chickpea flour (a small amount is low Fodmap)
4 tbsp white rice flour
12 tbsp tapioca flour
½ tsp salt
2 tsp dried oregano
¼ cup olive oil
2 eggs
3 tbsp grated Parmesan cheese

Instructions

1. Preheat oven to 180°C/350°F.
2. In a bowl, combine rice flakes, flours, salt and dried oregano. Mix well.
3. In another bowl lightly beat the eggs. Blend in the olive oil and cheese.
4. Combine wet and dry ingredients.
5. Knead the dough until well combined. If it is a little too wet, add some more rice flour; if it is a little too dry, add some water.
6. Between two sheets of baking paper, roll out the dough evenly and as thin as possible, to 1/8 -1/4"/0.5cm thickness.
7. Remove top paper. With a knife or pizza cutter, scour the dough into desired shapes but don't separate.
8. Transfer onto baking sheet (with bottom baking paper).
9. Bake for 12 minutes (depending on thickness of the crackers) or until edges turn golden brown.
10. Remove from the oven and let cool.
11. Break crackers at pre-cut edges. Serve fresh.

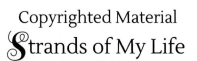

Strands of My Life

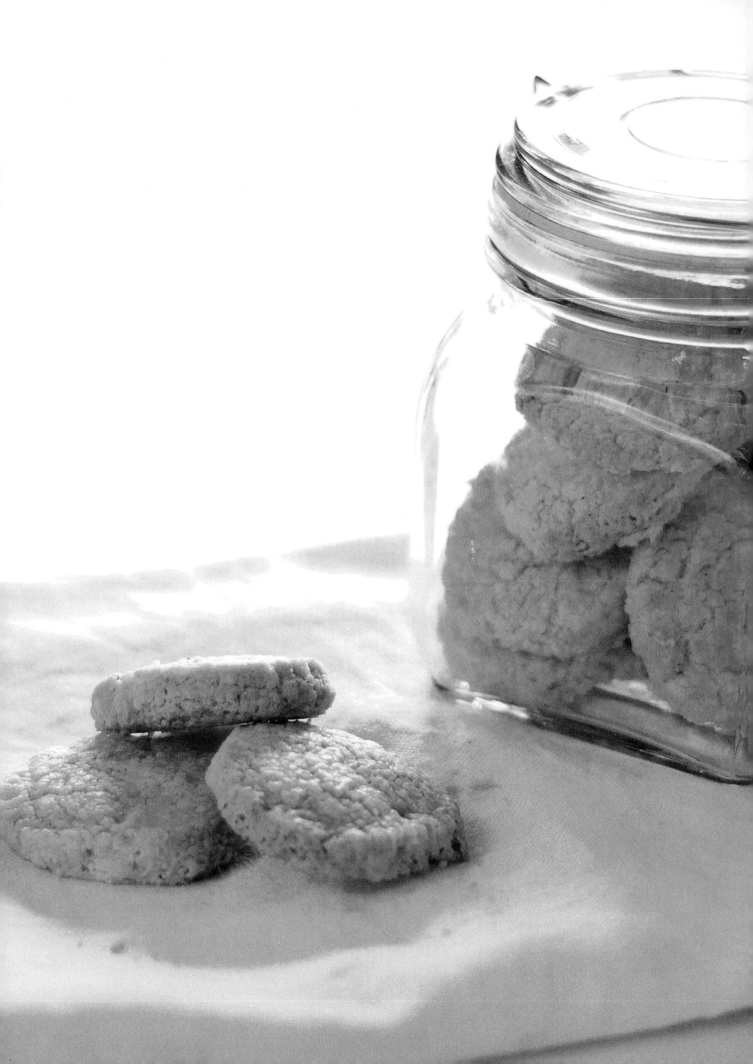

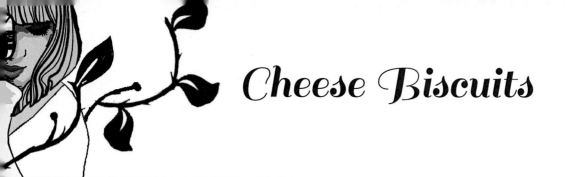

Cheese Biscuits

Ingredients

55gms/2oz white rice flour
30gms/1oz tapioca flour
25 gms/0.88oz potato starch
75gms/2.65oz butter
125gms/4.4oz grated hard cheese
¾ tsp salt
¾ tsp pepper
2-3 tbsp cold water (if necessary)

Instructions

1. Preheat the oven to 170°C/325°F.
2. Line a baking tray with baking paper.
3. Chop up the butter into small pieces.
4. Place the butter, flour, seasoning and cheese into a food processor and process until fine crumbs form.
5. Add a little water a bit at a time if necessary for it to form a dough.
6. Roll into a 12cm/4.75" long sausage, wrap in cling film and place in the fridge for 30 minutes.
7. Cut the roll into 1cm/1/3" slices and place on the baking tray.
8. Bake 10-15 minutes until golden.
9. Place on wire rack to cool.
10. Store in airtight container.

Strands of My Life

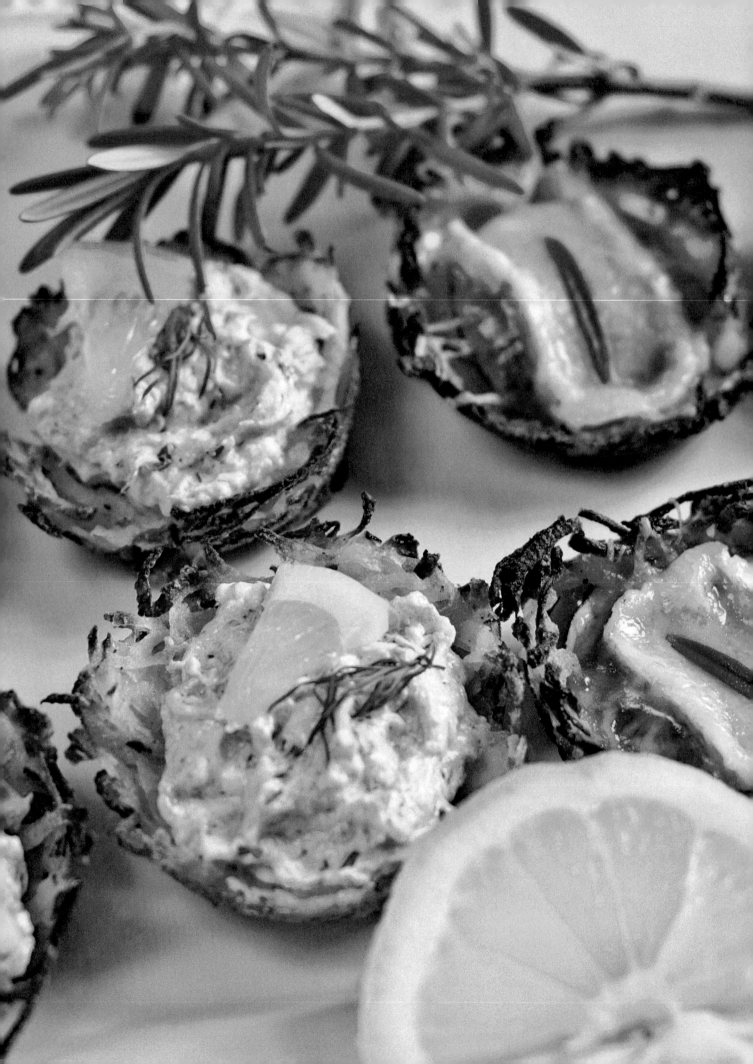

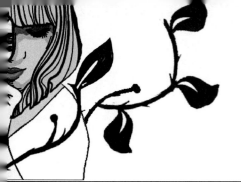

Rosti Pizzas

Ingredients

For the rosti:
4 potatoes
Rosemary
Olive Oil
Salt & pepper

For the salmon filling:
Cooked salmon fillet
Cream cheese (a small amount is low Fodmap)
Plain lactose-free yoghurt
Lemon juice
Dill, chopped
Salt & pepper

For the pizza filling:
Zucchini
Camembert
Tomato puree
Parmesan
Salt & pepper

Instructions

For the rosti:
1. Heat oven to 180°C/350°F.
2. Grate the potatoes and squeeze out all the liquid.
3. Mix in a bowl with a little olive oil and season it.
4. Chop up the rosemary very finely (not too much because it is quite strong) and add to the potatoes and mix well.
5. Oil large muffin tins.
6. Press the potato mixture into the pans to create little cups.
7. Bake in the oven until crispy though the inside will stay a little soft.
8. Cover with tin foil if the edges are getting too brown.

For the salmon filling:
1. Flake the salmon and mix all the ingredients to taste.
2. Place in the cooked rosti cups and serve.

For the pizza filling:
1. Slice up the zucchini to create one round per pizza and place it in the base of each one.
2. Place a small amount of tomato puree on top and season.
3. Slice up the Camembert and place a square on top of the puree.
4. Grate a little Parmesan over the top.
5. Place back in the oven for about 5 minutes until the cheese is melted. Eat warm.

Strands of My Life

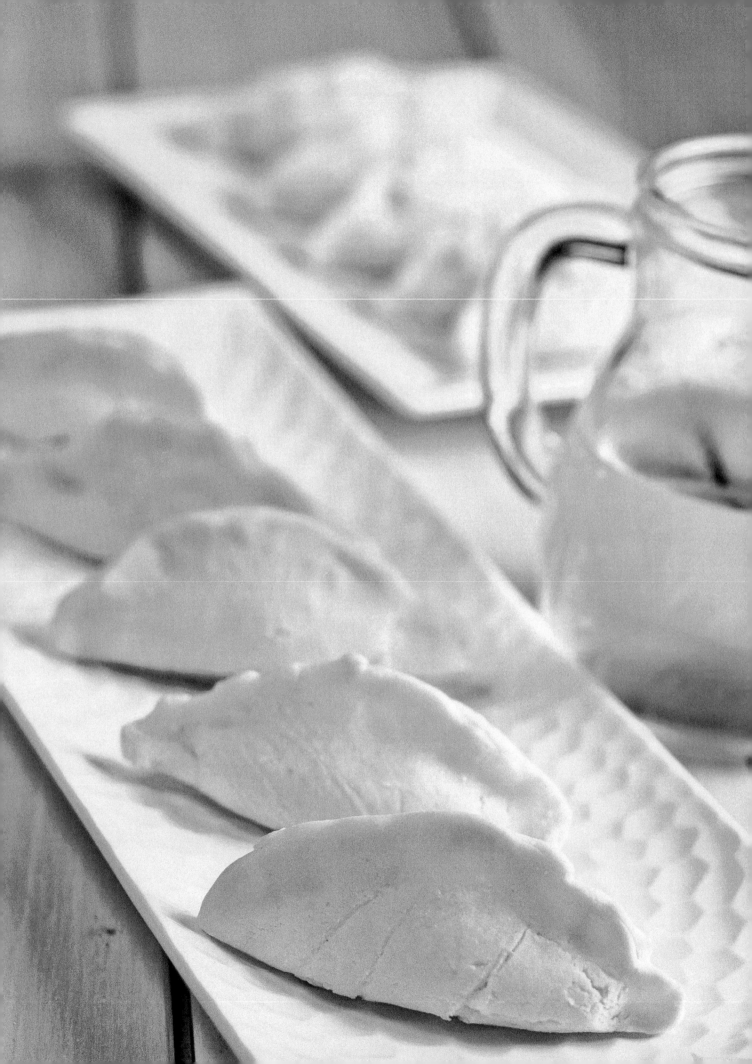

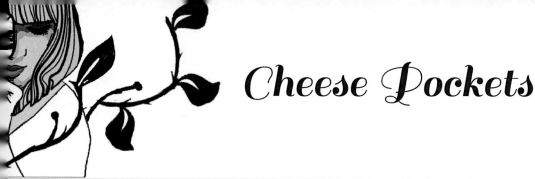

Cheese Pockets

Ingredients

For the pastry:
1.25 cups white rice flour
¾ cup tapioca flour
½ tsp baking powder
½ tsp salt
30gms/1 oz butter
¾ cup + 1 tbsp water

For the filling:
12gms/0.4oz melted butter
50gms/1.8oz grated cheese
1 egg
Salt
Pinch of cayenne
Juice of ½ lemon

Instructions

For the pastry:
1. Heat oven to 180°C/350°F.
2. Put all the dry ingredients in a food processor.
3. Add the butter and process.
4. Add the water slowly until a dough is formed.
5. Roll it out between two sheets of baking paper until it is thin but not too thin or it will break and the cheese mixture will ooze through.
6. Cut out rounds of the pastry and place a small amount of the filling in the centre.
7. Gently pull up the edges and create a wonton shape by pinching the edges together. There is no gluten so the pastry can be fragile - treat with respect.
8. Line a baking tray with baking paper and place the pockets on top.
9. Bake for 13 minutes.
10. Serve hot.

For the filling:
1. Mix everything together.

Strands of My Life

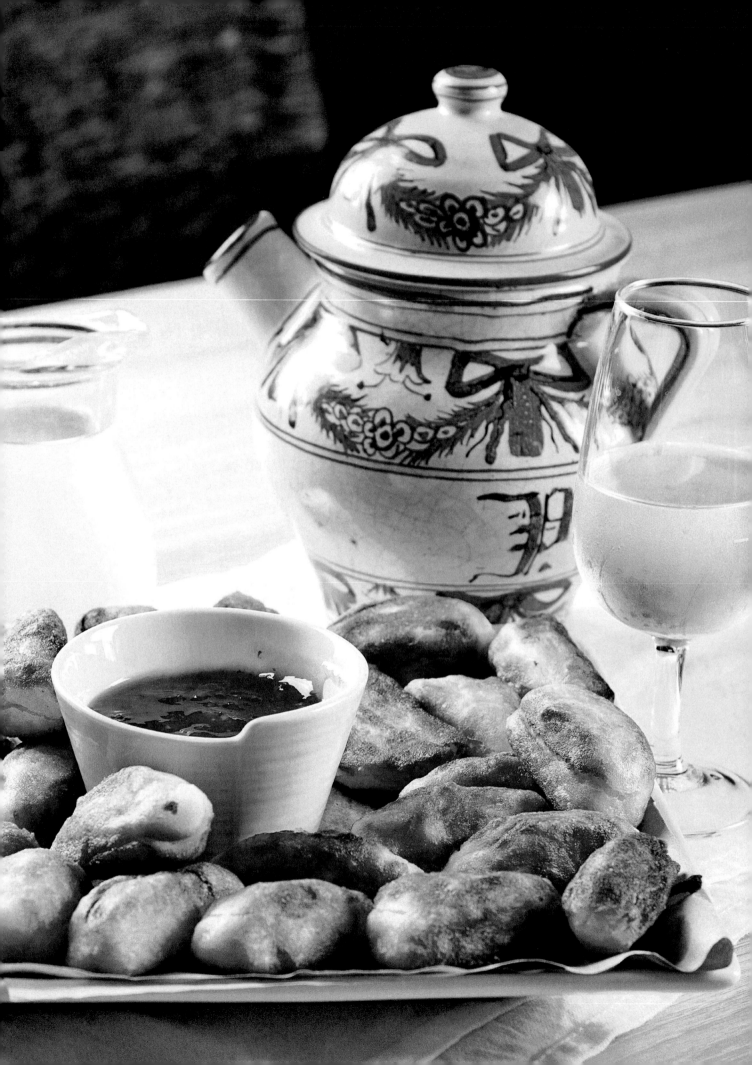

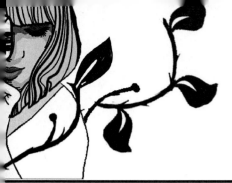

Fried Cheese Gnocchi Appetizers

Ingredients

500gms/17.5oz mashed potatoes
175 gms/6oz white rice flour
2 egg yolks
1 tsp salt
1 tsp grated ginger
100gms/3.5oz feta or hard cheese

Instructions

1. Place all ingredients except the cheese in a food processor and process until smooth.
2. Separate out into four pieces and roll each piece out into a long sausage.
3. Cut into 1"/2.5cm pieces.
4. Flatten them out into a circle with your fingers.
5. Place a piece of cheese on top of half of them.
6. Place the other halves over the top, squeeze the edges together and roll into ovals.
7. Boil a big pot of water and place the ovals in a few at a time so the water keeps boiling.
8. When they rise to the top, scoop them out and drain them well.
9. Heat oil in a pan and fry them on all sides until golden.
10. Drain on absorbent paper and eat while hot with a little hot (garlic-free) chilli sauce.

Strands of My Life

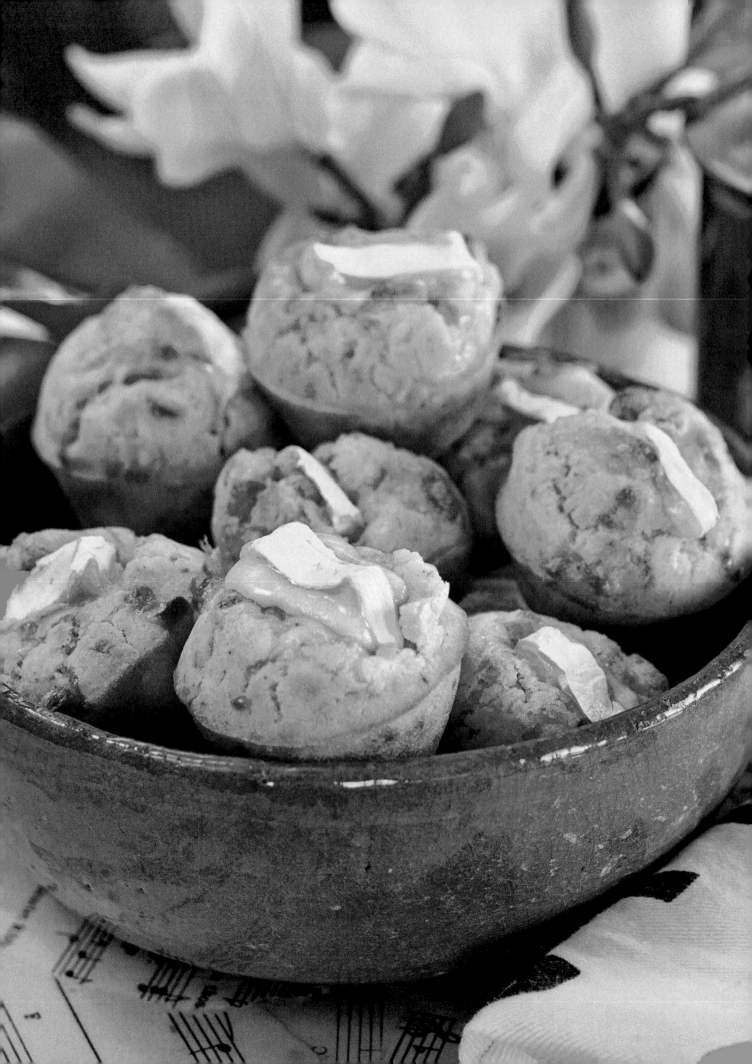

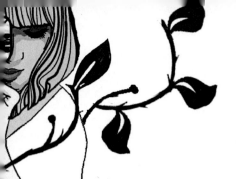

Camembert Mini Muffins

Ingredients

1.3 cups white rice flour
0.3 cup tapioca flour
0.3 cup potato starch
2 tsp baking powder
Pinch of salt
1 tsp paprika
1/2 tsp ground black pepper
1 tbsp fresh coriander, chopped
50gms/1.8oz butter
1 cup grated hard cheese
1.5 cups lactose-free milk
1 egg
250gms/8.8oz Camembert

Instructions

1. Heat oven to 180°C/350°F.
2. Sift the flours, baking powder, paprika and salt together.
3. Rub the butter into the dry ingredients.
4. Add the pepper, coriander and grated cheese.
5. Beat the egg and milk together and add to the mixture.
6. Butter or oil a mini muffin tin and fill each compartment almost to the top.
7. Bake for 12 minutes.
8. Remove from the heat, slice a small cut in each muffin and place a thin slice of Camembert in the cut.
9. Place back in the oven for 3 minutes.
10. Serve warm to enjoy the melted Camembert.

Makes 24

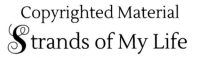

Strands of My Life

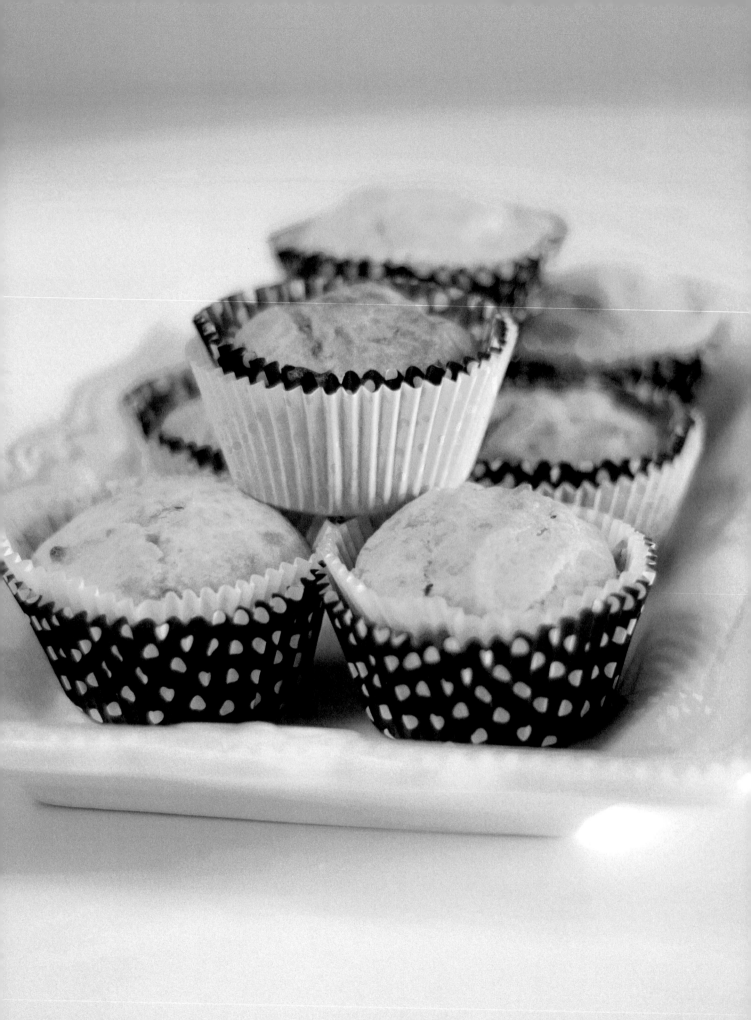

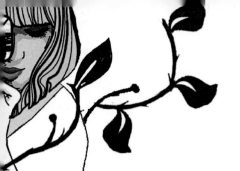

Potato & Cheese Muffins

Ingredients

250gms/8.8oz cooked mashed potato
1 cup water
1 cup oil
2 eggs
1.3 cups white rice flour
1/3 cup tapioca flour
1/3 cup potato starch
2 tsp baking powder
pinch of salt
1 tsp paprika
¼ tsp black pepper
1 tbsp parsley

Instructions

1. Heat oven to 180°C/350°F
2. Place the potato, water, eggs and oil in a food processor and blend well.
3. Sift the dry ingredients together.
4. Add the wet ingredients to the dry.
5. Stir in the grated cheese and parsley and mix well.
6. Place cupcake papers into a 12 capacity muffin tin.
7. Lightly spray them with oil.
8. Spoon the mixture into the cupcake papers.
9. Place in the oven for about 20 minutes until a skewer comes out clean.
10. Remove from the oven and cool them down on a cooling rack.
11. Eat fresh or freeze for another day.

Strands of My Life

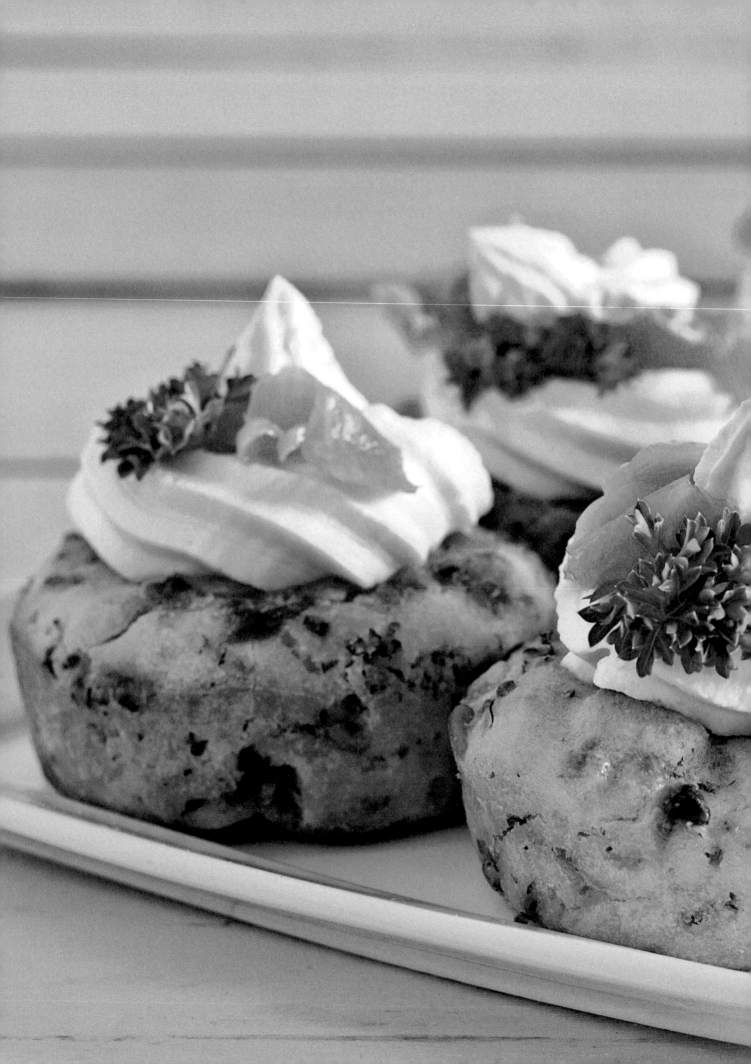

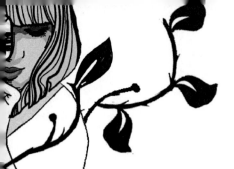

Cheese & Parsley Muffins

Ingredients

153gms/5oz white rice flour
22gms/0.8oz tapioca flour
45gms/1.6oz potato starch
150gms/5oz polenta
½ tsp salt
½ tsp sugar
4 tbsp chopped parsley
½ cup toasted pine nuts
1 cup grated mozzarella cheese
450mls/16 fl oz lactose-free milk
4 tbsp olive oil
2 eggs, beaten

Instructions

1. Heat oven to 180°C/350°F.
2. Grease a 12-capacity muffin baking tin.
3. Combine the dry ingredients well including the cheese, pine nuts and parsley.
4. Whisk together the wet ingredients.
5. Add the wet to the dry and combine.
6. Spoon into the muffin tins and bake for 15-20 minutes.
7. Garnish them with a swirl of cream cheese (a little is low Fodmap).
8. Eat fresh or freeze for another day without the cream cheese.

Strands of My Life

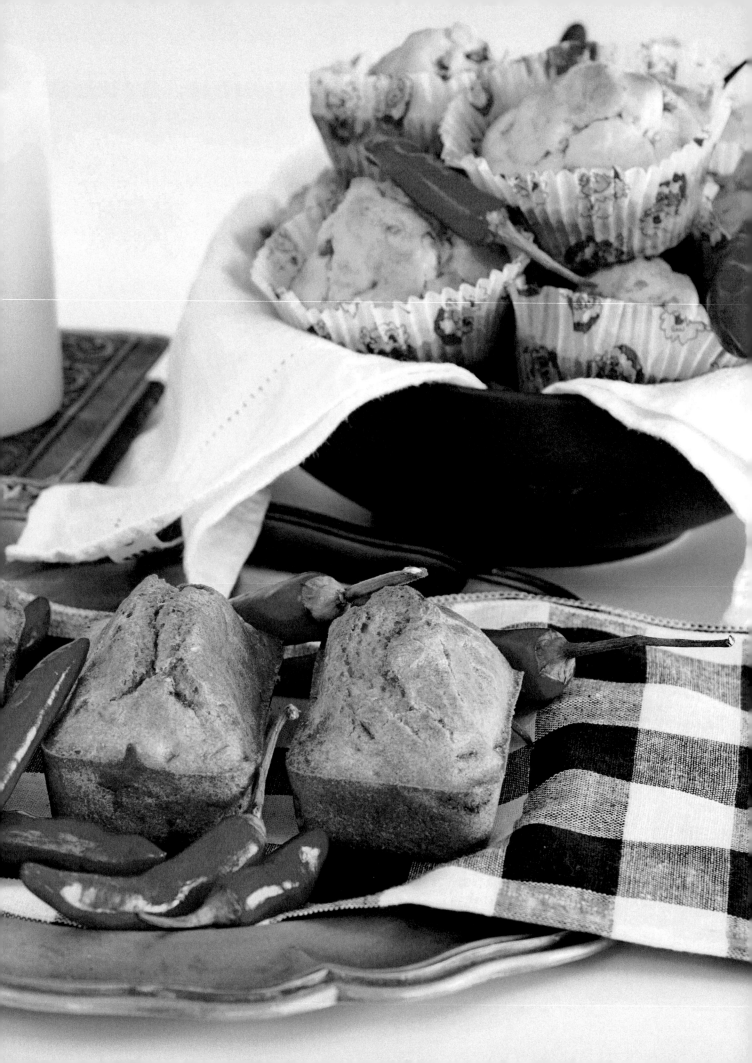

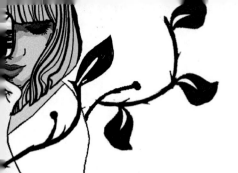

Savoury Vegetable Muffins

Ingredients

40gms/1.4oz buckwheat flour
40gms/1.4oz brown rice flour
80gms/2.8oz potato starch
2 teaspoons baking powder
4 eggs
120gms/4.2oz lactose-free milk
60gms/2.1oz grated parmesan cheese
80mls/2.7oz extra virgin olive oil
1 tsp salt
Pepper
2 fresh red chilies
1 tsp grated fresh ginger
300gms/10.6oz mixture of chopped eggplant, carrots, boiled potatoes & zucchini

Instructions

1. Heat oven to 180°C/350°F.
2. Chop all the vegetables including the chillis finely.
3. Heat a teaspoon of rice bran oil in a frying pan and cook the vegetables and ginger until they are softened. Season a little.
4. Separate the eggs.
5. Add the olive oil to the egg yolks slowly as if you were making a mayonnaise so that it all amalgamates well to form a cream.
6. Sift the dry ingredients together.
7. Add them slowly, alternating with the milk, to the yolk mixture.
8. Add the cheese.
9. Beat the egg whites until they are stiff and fold into the mixture along with the cooked vegetables. (Make sure there is no liquid with the vegetables.)
10. Grease a 12-mould muffin tin or mini loaf tins and spoon the mixture in.
11. Bake for around 20 minutes for the muffin tins and 30 minutes for the mini loaf tins. Check that a skewer comes out clean.
12. Leave to cool a little and then tip them out onto a cooling rack.
13. Eat warm or cold and freeze the leftovers.

Strands of My Life

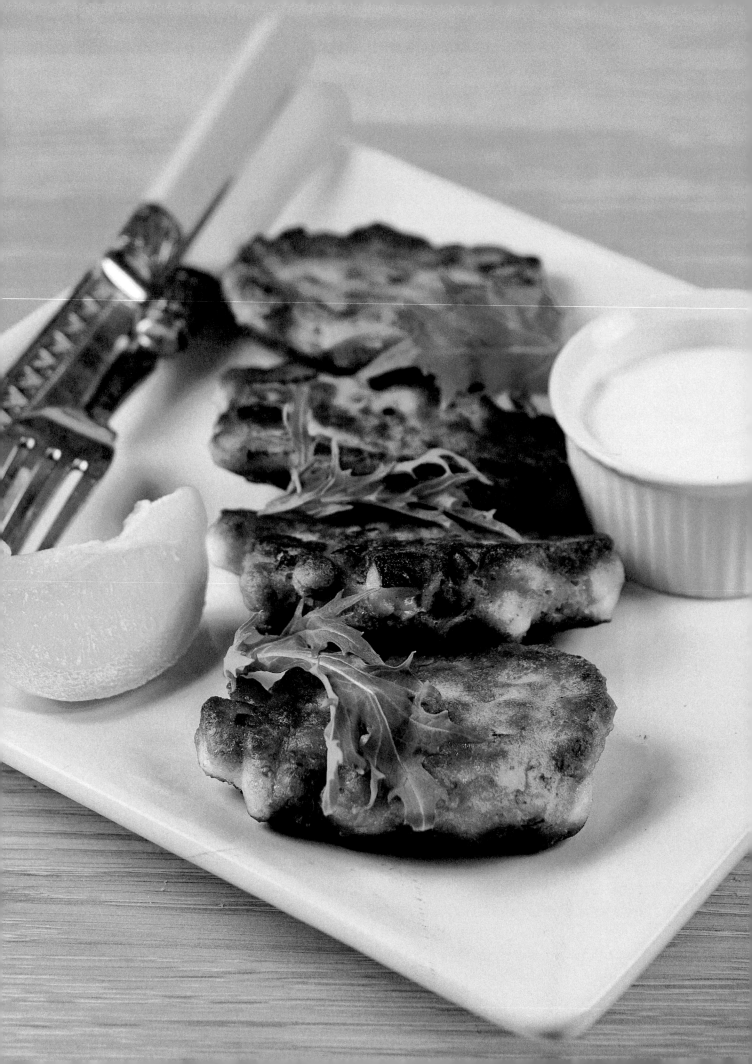

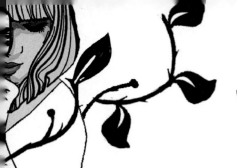

Haloumi & Pea Fritters

Ingredients

1 cup peas, fresh or frozen (thawed)
1 tbsp of butter
1 tsp garlic-infused oil
3 spring onions, green part only, finely sliced
2 zucchini, diced
200gms/7oz haloumi cheese, diced 1cm pieces
olive oil for cooking fritters

For the batter:
1/2 cup white rice flour
1/4 cup tapioca flour
1 tsp sea salt
1/4 cup chopped mint
1/2 tsp tumeric
1 tsp ground cumin
Pinch chili flakes
3 eggs

Instructions

1. Melt the butter and oil in a pan and cook the spring onions and zucchini with the salt for 4 minutes.
2. Add the peas and cook 1 minute. Cool.
3. Put all the batter ingredients in a food processor and blend until smooth.
4. Stir the cooled vegetables and haloumi into the batter.
5. Heat a little olive oil in a pan and cook small spoonfuls of mixture for 2-3 minutes each side until golden and cooked through.
6. Place the fritters in a warm oven until they are all cooked.
7. Arrange the fritters on a plate and serve with a bowl of thick plain lactose-free yoghurt.

Note: 1/4 cup peas and 2 slices haloumi are low Fodmap

Strands of My Life

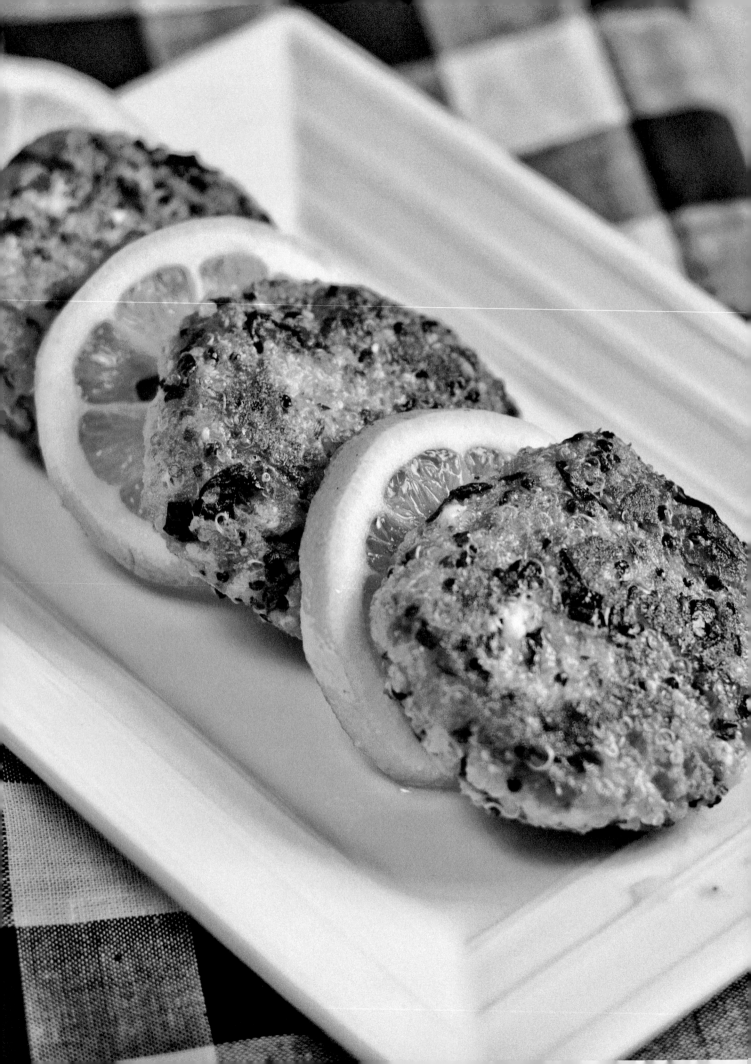

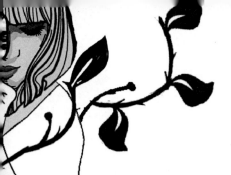

Feta & Quinoa Patties

Ingredients

1.25 cups quinoa
1 leek (green part only)
2 tbsp fresh coriander
1 tbsp fresh mint
Zest of ½ lemon
200gms/7 oz feta
100gms/3.5oz spinach
2 eggs
1.5 cups dry gluten-free breadcrumbs
Salt & pepper

Instructions

1. Cook the quinoa according to the packet instructions.
2. Finely chop the leek, spinach and herbs. Put into a bowl.
3. Add the lemon zest.
4. Dice the feta and add.
5. Make sure the water has cooked off the quinoa and that it is relatively dry.
6. Add to the mixture with the breadcrumbs.
7. Break in the eggs and season with salt and pepper.
8. Mix everything well.
9. Form into patties and fry in a little oil until browned on both sides.

Note: Makes 18 patties

Strands of My Life

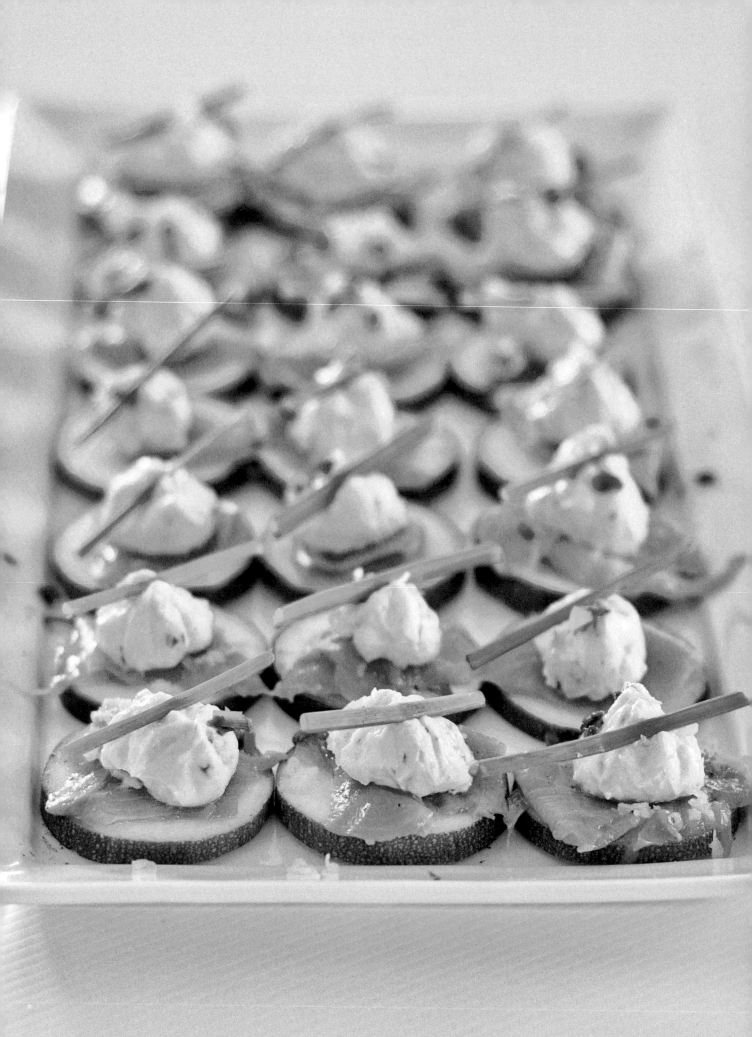

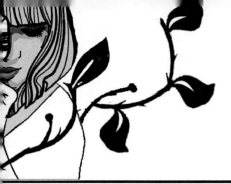

Salmon Cottage Cheese Bites

Ingredients

Two fat zucchini
150g/5.3oz cottage cheese
100g/3.5oz smoked salmon
Zest of 1 lemon
½ tsp wasabi
1 tbsp coconut milk
Chives
Salt & pepper

Instructions

1. Slice the zucchini into thin rounds and lay out on a large plate
2. Place a small slice of salmon on each one.
3. Sprinkle with some chopped chives
4. Place the cottage cheese, most of the lemon zest, the wasabi, milk, a pinch of salt and a grinding of pepper in a small food processor and process until smooth.
5. Pipe onto the salmon.
6. Sprinkle with more chives and the rest of the lemon zest.

Strands of My Life

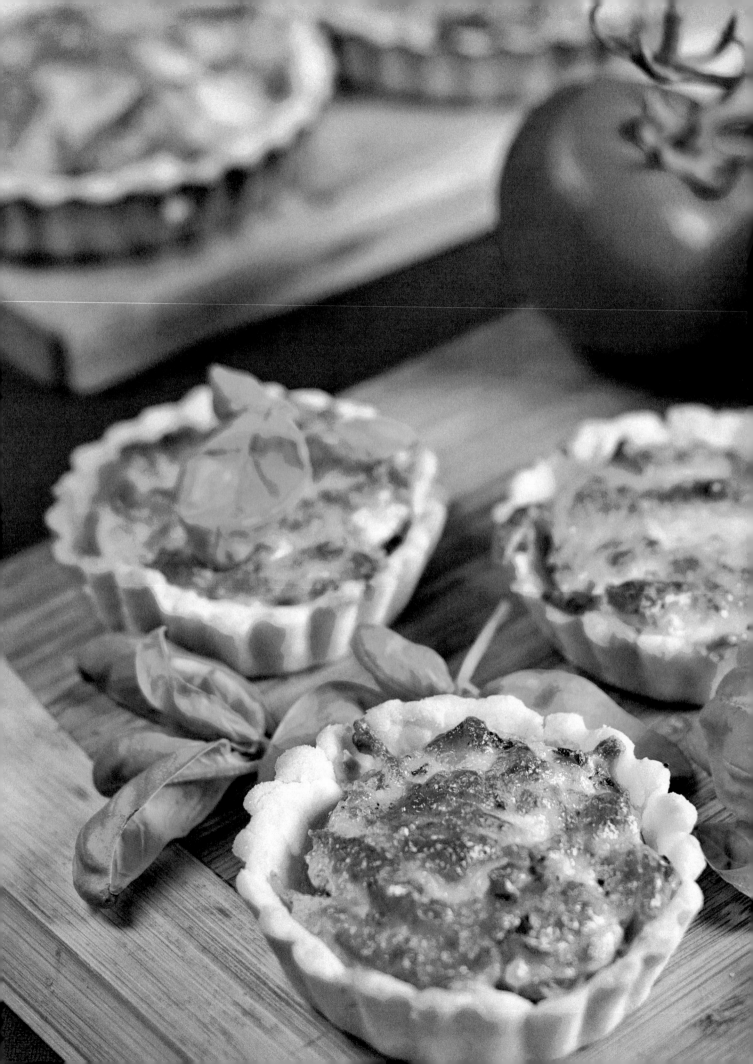

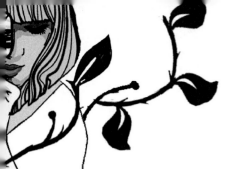

Basil & Tomato Tartlets

Ingredients

For the pastry:
133gms/4.7oz white rice flour
22gms/0.8oz tapioca flour
45gms/1.6oz potato starch
Pinch of salt
100gms/3.5oz butter
1 medium egg

For the filling:
5 cups grated mozzarella
4 medium tomatoes
1 cup basil leaves
1 tsp garlic-infused oil
½ cup mayonnaise
¼ cup Parmesan cheese
Black pepper

For the mayonnaise:
1 egg
2 tbsp lemon juice
1/2 tsp salt
1.2 tsp pepper
1/2 tsp dry mustard
237mls/1/2 pt oil

Instructions

For the pastry:
1. Blend all the dry ingredients in a food processor.
2. Add the butter cut into small pieces to the food processor and process until fine crumbs form.
3. Add the egg and process until it forms a dough.
4. Remove from the processor and add a little more rice flour if it is too wet or water if it is too dry - this depends on the size of your egg.
5. Press out into greased tart tins and place in the fridge for 30 minutes.
6. Preheat the oven to 180°C/350°F.
7. Place baking paper in the base of the tarts and fill with rice or dried beans and blind bake for 15 minutes.

For the filling:
8. Sprinkle ½ cup of mozzarella cheese on the hot bases.
9. Cut the tomatoes into thin wedges and arrange on the top of the cheese.
10. Place the basil in a food processor and chop finely.
11. Add the oil and whiz again.
12. Sprinkle this mixture over the tomatoes.
13. Place all the mayonnaise ingredients except the oil into a blender and mix together.
14. Pour in the oil slowly while continuing to blend.
15. Add the remaining cheese, parmesan and pepper to the mayonnaise.
16. Spoon this mixture evenly over the basil.
17. Bake in the oven for 10-15 minutes. Watch the tops don't brown too much.
18. Serve hot.

Strands of My Life

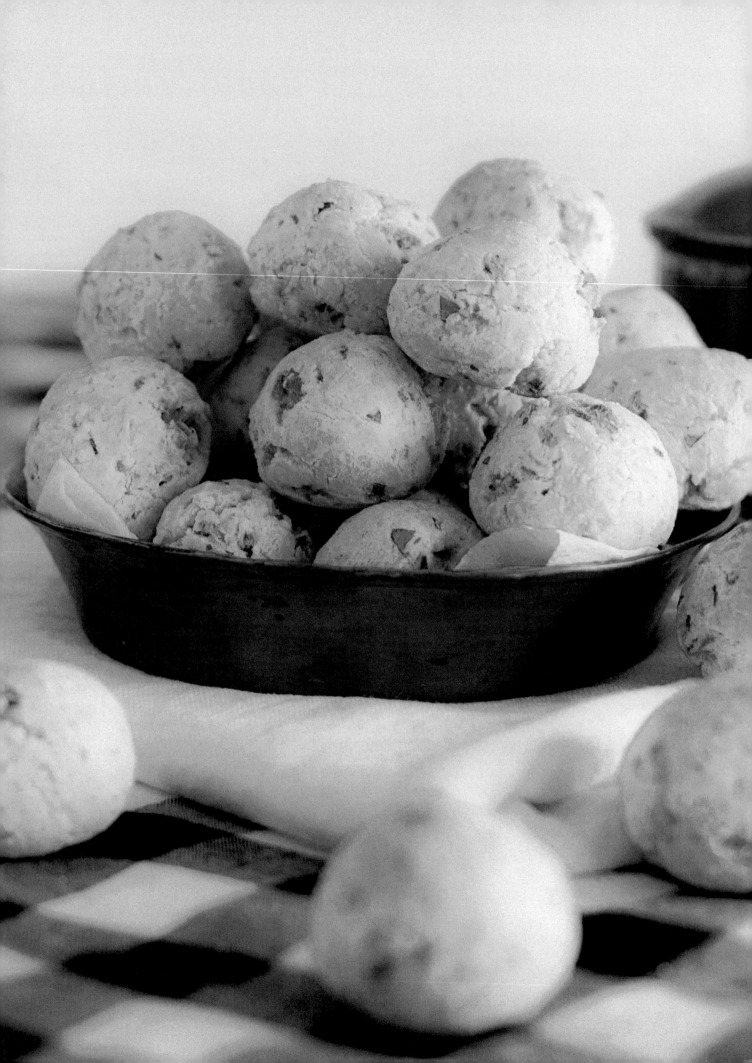

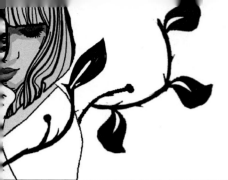

Mini Chicken Bread Rolls

Ingredients

1/3 cup rice bran oil
1/3 cup water
1/3 cup rice milk
Pinch of salt
3/4 cup tapioca flour
1 cup white rice flour
1/2 cup potato starch
2 eggs
1 cup chopped chicken cooked
1 tbsp chopped parsley

Instructions

1. Heat oven to 180°C/350°F.
2. Combine the flours and salt in a bowl.
3. Heat the oil, milk and water in a saucepan until almost boiling.
4. Add the hot liquid to the flour mixture and stir together.
5. Add the eggs and mix well.
6. Add the chicken, parsley and sundried chicken.
7. Roll small balls from the mixture and place on an oven tray covered by baking paper.
8. Bake for about 20 minutes until browned.
9. Serve while warm.

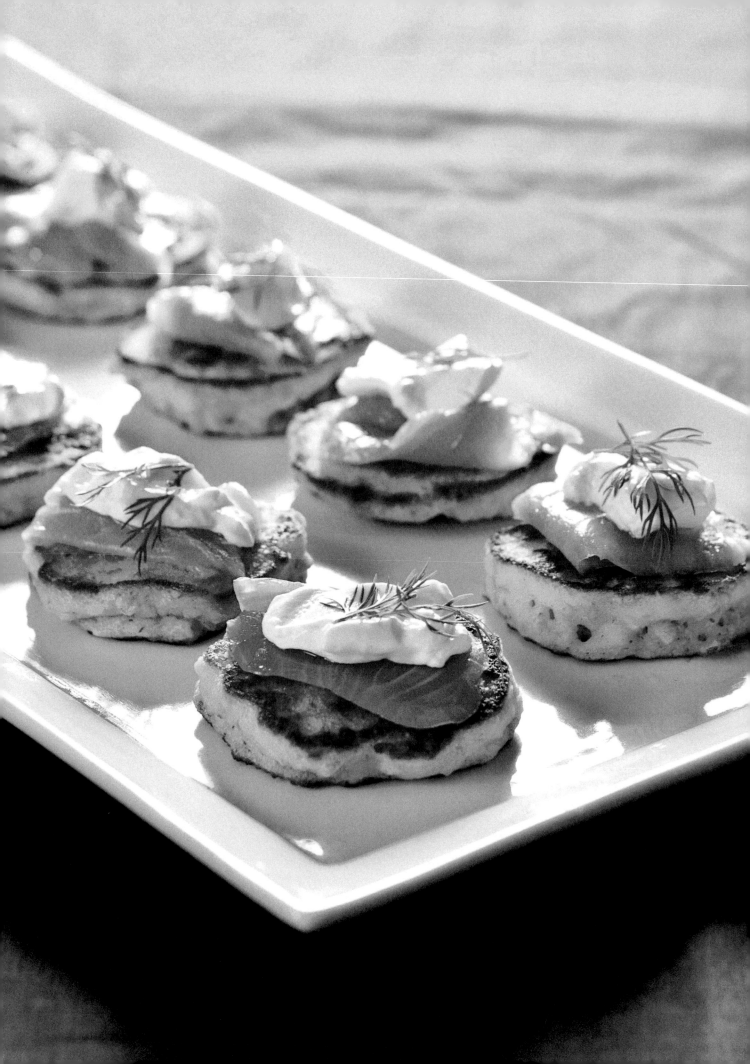

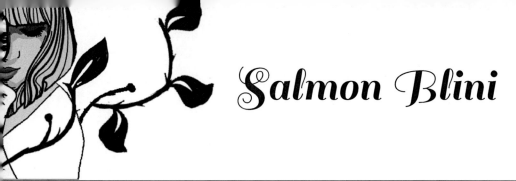

Salmon Blini

Ingredients

83gms/3oz white rice flour
21gms/0.75oz tapioca flour
21gms/0.75oz potato starch
Pinch of salt
1 egg
1 cup milk

Instructions

1. Sift the flours and salt together.
2. Add the lightly beaten egg and mix as well as possible.
3. Add the milk slowly mixing well in between additions.
4. Melt a little butter in a frying pan and add tablespoons of mixture to the pan, leaving a space between each one.
5. When bubbles form all over the pancake mixture, flip them over and cook on the other side.
6. Repeat with all the mixture.
7. Serve with smoked salmon, lactose-free yoghurt and a little dill.

Strands of My Life

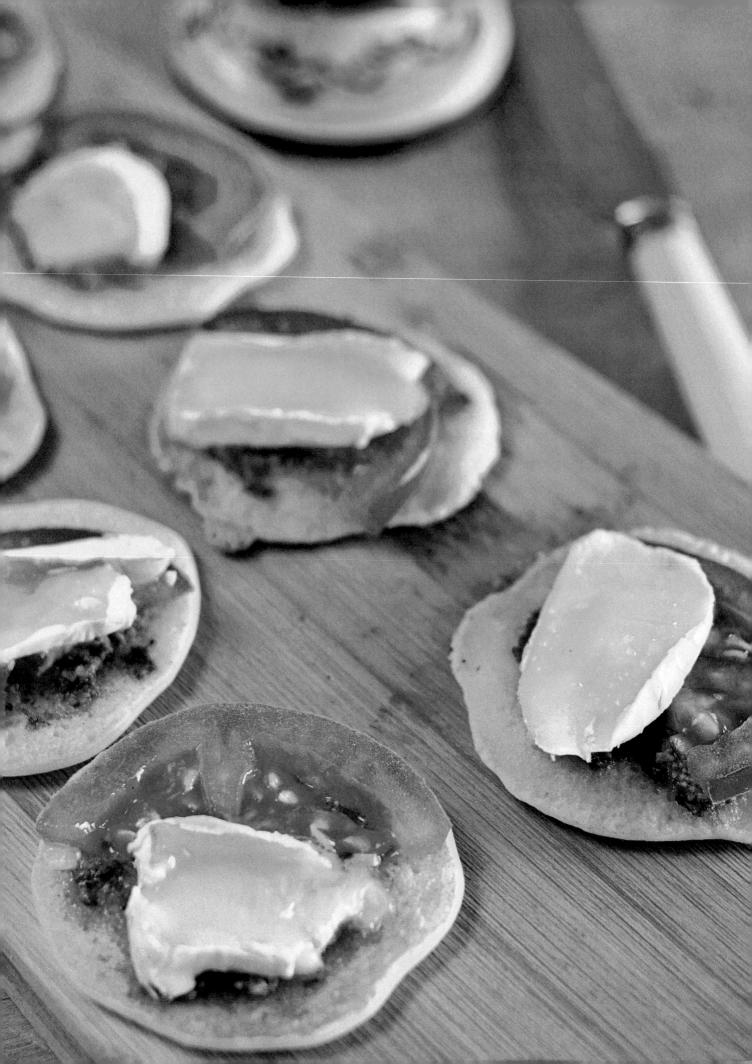

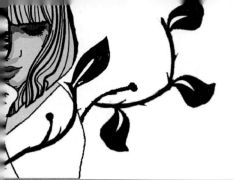

Tomato Pesto Nibbles

Ingredients

83gms/3oz white rice flour
21gms/0.75oz tapioca flour
21gms/0.75oz potato starch
Pinch of salt
1 cup milk

Topping:
Tomatoes
Pesto sauce
Camembert cheese

Instructions

1. Sift the flours and salt together.
2. Add the milk slowly mixing well in between additions.
3. Melt a little butter in a frying pan and add tablespoons of mixture to the pan, leaving a space between each one.
4. When bubbles form all over the pancake mixture, flip them over and cook on the other side.
5. At this stage, smear a little pesto on the cooked side and place half a slice of tomato and a thin wedge of camembert on top.
6. Let them cook until the undersides are brown and the cheese softened.
7. Repeat with all the mixture.
8. Serve warm.

Makes 12

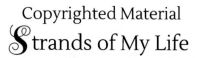
Strands of My Life

SWEET SNACKS

———— * ————

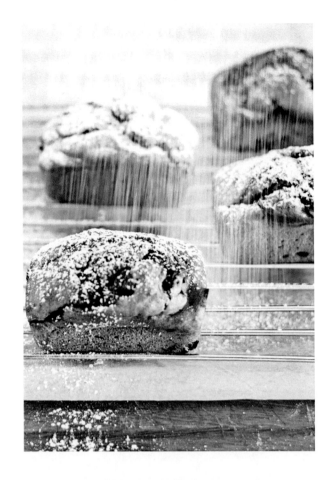

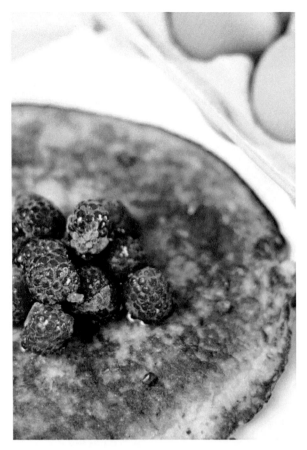

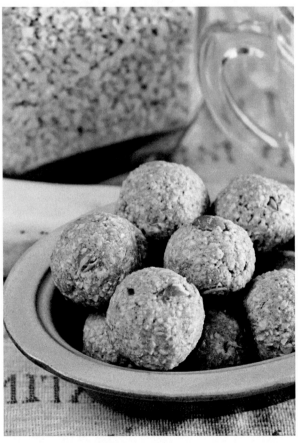

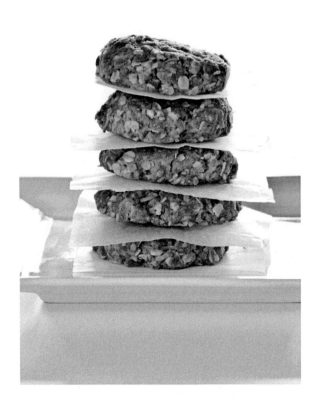

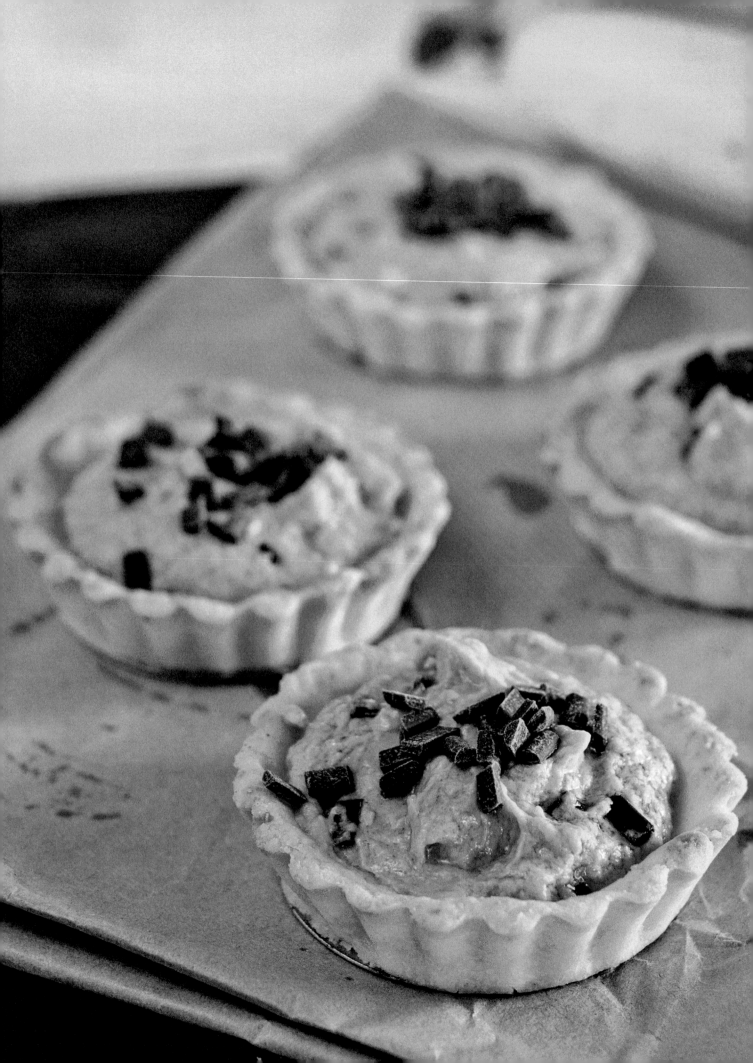

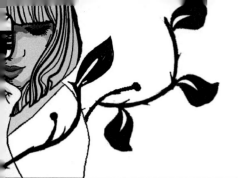

Peanut Butter Banana Tarts

Ingredients

For the pastry shell:
133gms/4.7oz white rice flour
22gms/0.8oz tapioca flour
45gms/1.6oz potato starch
Pinch of salt
1 tbsp sugar
100gms/3.5oz butter
1 medium egg

For the Filling:
1 banana
1 cup smooth peanut butter
1/2 cup plain lactose-free Greek yoghurt
1/4 cup dark chocolate chips

Instructions

For the pastry:
1. Preheat the oven to 180°C/350°F.
2. Blend all the dry ingredients in a food processor.
3. Add the butter cut into small pieces to the food processor and process until fine crumbs form.
4. Add the egg and process until it forms a dough.
5. Add a little water if it is too dry - this depends on the size of your egg.
6. Remove from the processor and knead together.
7. Press out into small buttered tart tins.
8. Place baking paper in the base of the tart shells and fill with rice or dried beans and blind bake for 10 minutes, then remove the paper and beans/rice and cook for a further 4 minutes.
9. Remove from the oven and slide out of the tins and leave to cool completely.

For the Filling:
10. Place everything except the chocolate chips in a processor and process until smooth.
11. Place the mixture in a bowl and add the chocolate chips.
12. Pile the mixture into the cooked pastry shells and serve or place in the fridge.

Makes 10 small tarts

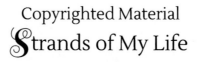
Strands of My Life

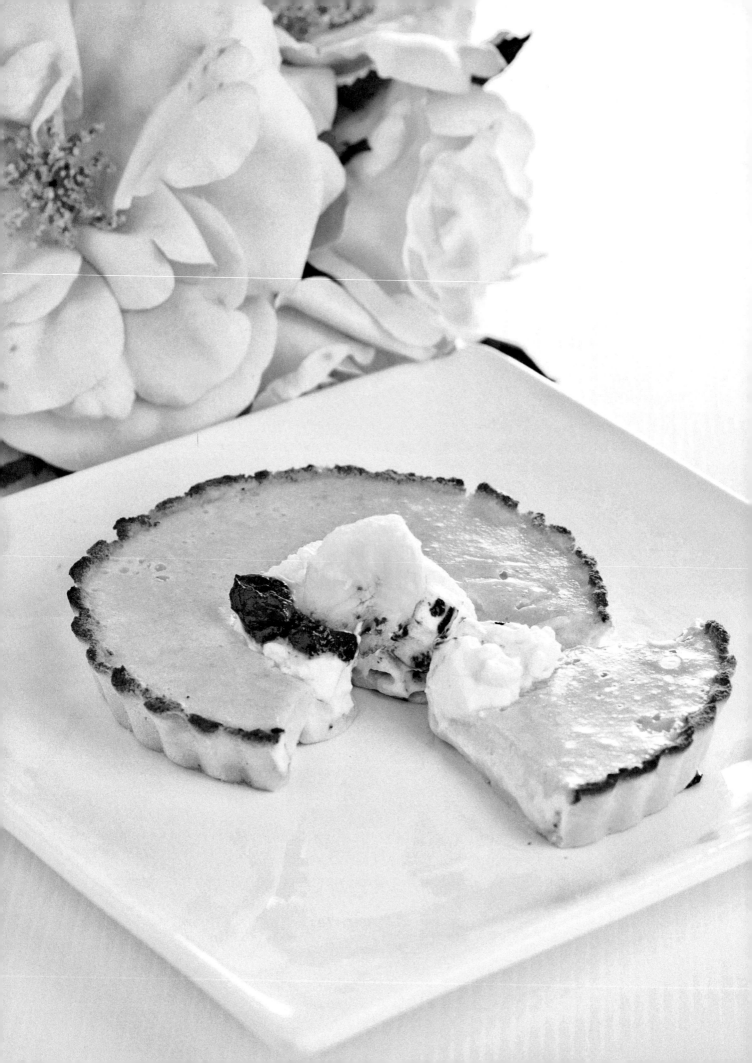

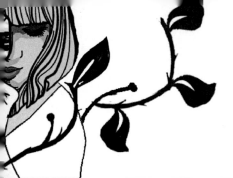

Banana Mousse Tarts

Ingredients

For the pastry shell:
133gms/4.7oz white rice flour
22gms/0.8oz tapioca flour
45gms/1.6oz potato starch
Pinch of salt
1 heaped tbsp sugar
100gms/3.5oz butter
1 medium egg

For the mousse:
3 bananas
300ml chilled coconut cream
2 tsp gelatin powder
150ml water

Instructions

For the pastry:
1. Preheat the oven to 180°C/350°F.
2. Blend all the dry ingredients in a food processor.
3. Add the butter cut into small pieces to the food processor and process until fine crumbs form.
4. Add the egg and process until it forms a dough.
5. Add a little water if it is too dry - this depends on the size of your egg.
6. Remove from the processor and knead together.
7. Press out into small buttered tart tins.
8. Place baking paper in the base of the tart shells and fill with rice or dried beans and blind bake for 10 minutes, then remove the paper and beans/rice and cook for a further 4 minutes.
9. Remove from the oven and slide out of the tins and leave to cool completely.

For the the mousse:
10. Heat the water in a small saucepan and add the gelatine to dissolve.
11. Process the bananas in a food processor until smooth.
12. Whip the coconut cream until firm.
13. Fold in the banana mixture.
14. Once the gelatin is completely dissolved, cool it a bit and then add to the banana cream.
15. Pour into the cooled pastry shells and refigerate.

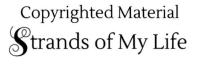

Strands of My Life

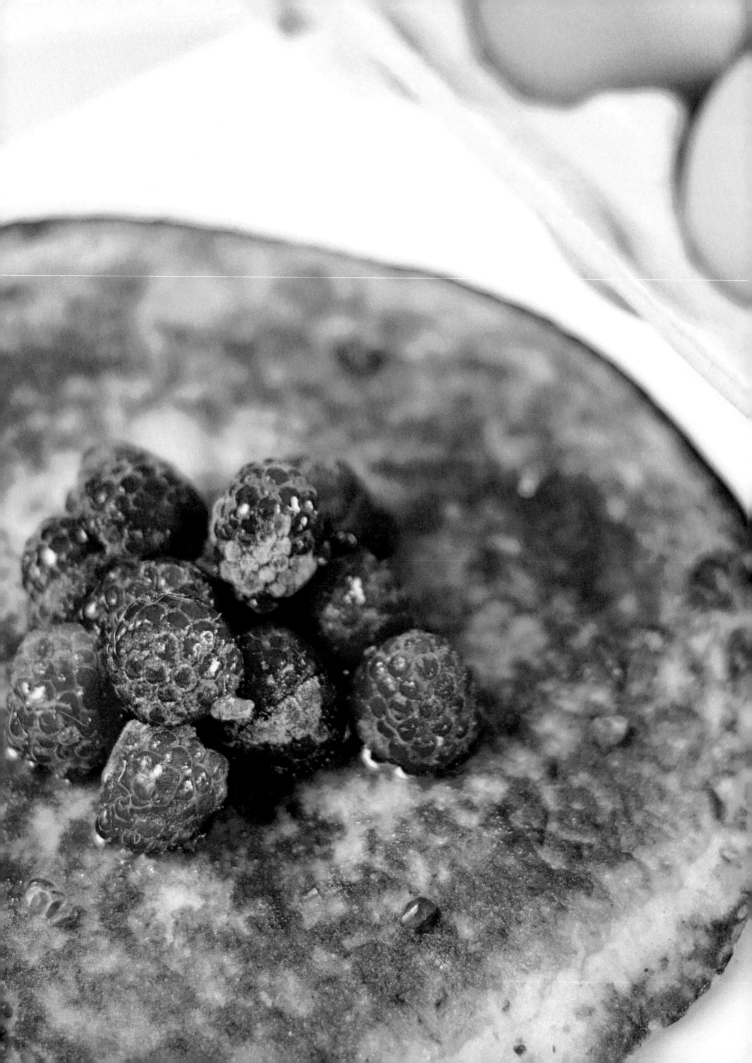

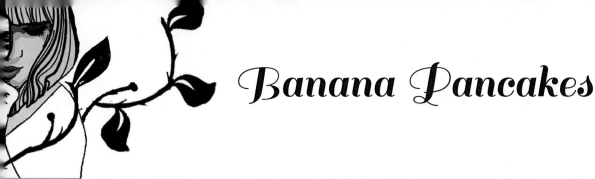

Banana Pancakes

Ingredients

1 banana
2 eggs
1 tsp vanilla essence
Butter
Maple syrup
10 raspberries

Instructions

1. Beat the eggs, bananas and vanilla essence together until well blended.
2. Melt a little butter in a frying pan.
3. Once it is bubbling, pour ½ the egg mixture into the pan.
4. Once it is set on one side, flip it over and cook on the other side.
5. Slip out onto a plate and keep warm.
6. Cook the rest of the pancake mixture in the same way,
7. Serve each with 5 raspberries and a little drizzle of maple syrup.

Makes 2 pancakes

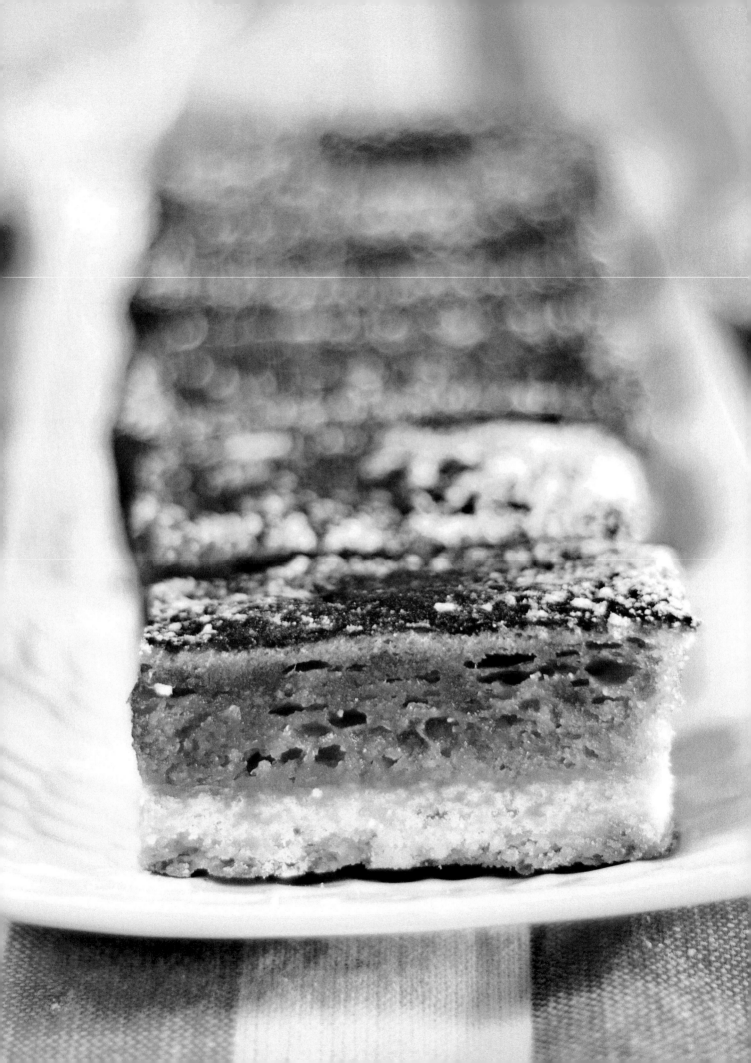

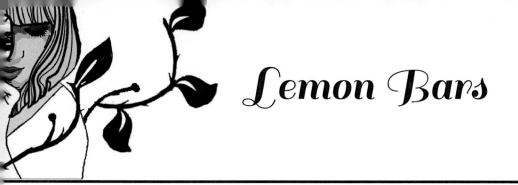

Lemon Bars

Ingredients

For the base:

1 cup butter
½ cup sugar
Pinch of salt
¾ cup rice flour
¼ cup potato starch
¼ cup tapioca flour

For the topping:

2 eggs
¾ cup cane sugar
1 tbsp rice flour
1 tbsp tapioca flour
½ tsp baking powder
6 tbsp lemon juice

Instructions

For the base:

1. Pre-heat the oven to 350°F/180°C.
2. Cream the butter and sugar together.
3. Sift the flours and salt together.
4. Mix the dry with the wet ingredients.
5. Press into a buttered 20cm/8" baking dish.
6. Bake for 25-30 minutes.

For the topping:

1. Place everything in a food processor to mix well together.
2. Pour over the baked but still hot base.
3. Place back in the oven for 15-20 minutes.
4. Remove from the oven and cool before cutting into bars.

Strands of My Life

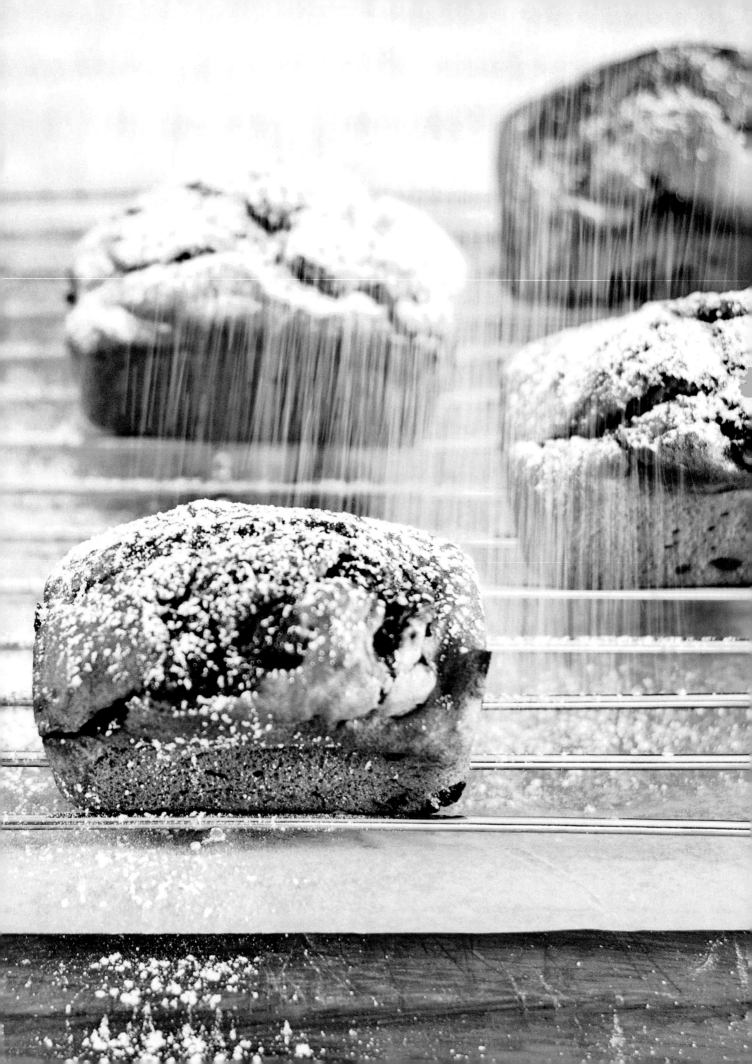

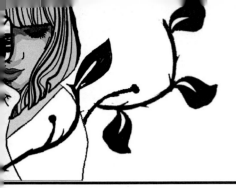

Blueberry & Raspberry Mini Loaves

Ingredients

1 ripe banana
1 medium potato boiled and mashed
57gms/2 oz melted unsalted butter
1 tsp almond essence
2 eggs
½ cup brown sugar
1/3 cup white rice flour
1/3 cup brown rice flour
¼ cup tapioca flour
¼ cup potato starch
1 tsp cinnamon
1 tsp baking powder
½ tsp baking soda
pinch of salt
¾ cup blueberries (fresh or frozen)
½ cup raspberries (fresh or frozen)

Instructions

1. Heat oven to 180°C/350°F.
2. In a food processor, blend the banana, potato, butter and almond essence.
3. Add the eggs and blend again.
4. Sift all the dry ingredients together.
5. Add the dry ingredients to the wet and mix well.
6. Add the berries and mix gently.
7. Pour the mixture into mini loaf tins and bake for 20 minutes.
8. Cool before eating but eat them fresh or freeze them.

Strands of My Life

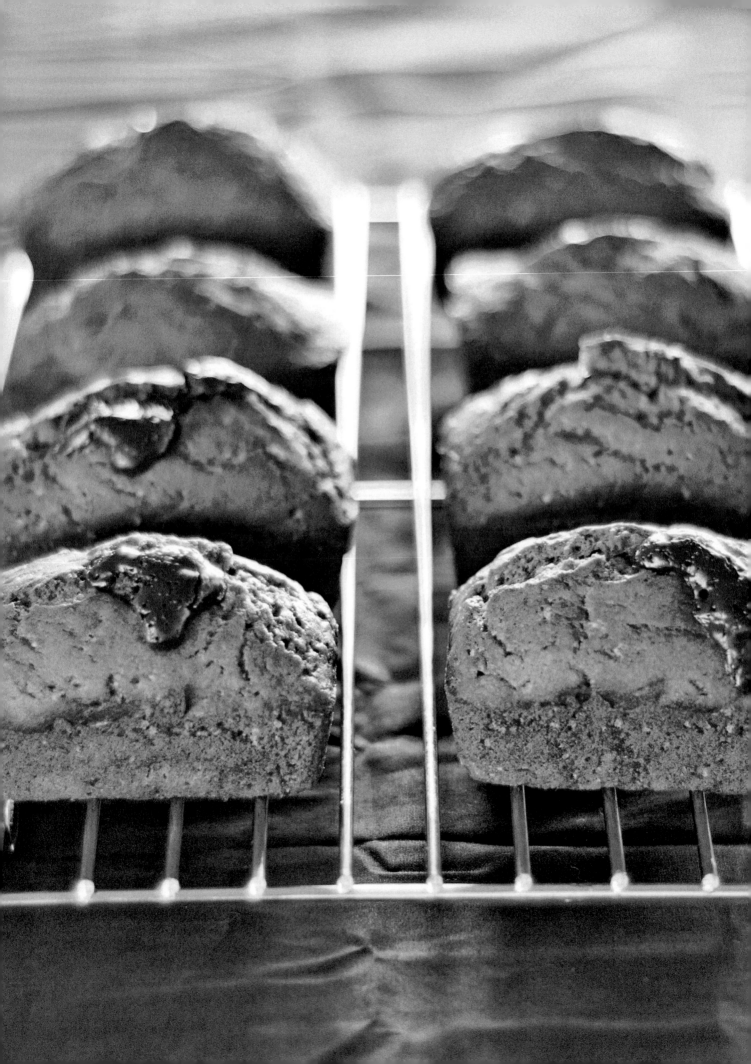

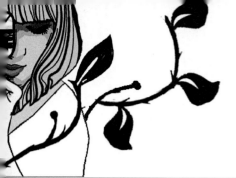

Mini Banana & Chocolate Loaves

Ingredients

2 ripe bananas
57gms/2oz butter, melted
2 eggs
1 tsp vanilla essence
2/3 cup white rice flour
3 tbsp tapioca flour
3 tbsp potato starch
1 tsp cinnamon
1 tsp baking powder
1/2 tsp baking soda
1/2 cup cane sugar
Pinch of salt
A small block of 70% dark chocolate

Instructions

1. Preheat oven to 350°F/180°C.
2. Butter or oil 8 mini loaf tins.
3. Place the first 4 ingredients in a food processor and process until smooth.
4. Sift the next 7 ingredients together and mix with a whisk.
5. Add the sugar and mix.
6. Add the wet ingredients to the dry and blend well to incorporate some air.
7. Place half the mixture evenly into the tins.
8. Break up the chocolate and place some pieces on top of the batter in each tin.
9. Fill the tins with the remaining batter.
10. Bake for 15 minutes or until a skewer comes out clean

Strands of My Life

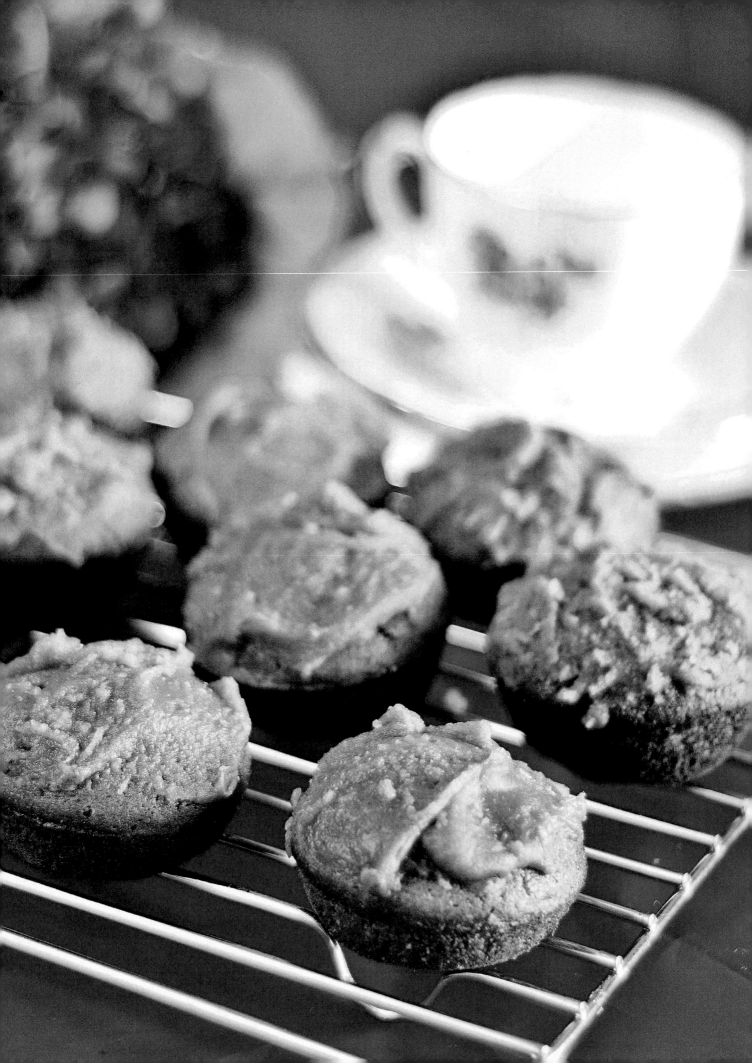

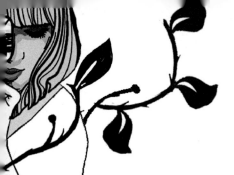

Ginger & Potato Muffins

Ingredients

For the muffins:
2 eggs
¾ cup sugar
1 cup coconut oil
¾ cup golden syrup
2 tsp ginger
1 tsp cinnamon
½ tsp baking soda
1.3 cups white rice flour
1/3 cup tapioca flour
1/3 cup potato starch
2 tsp baking powder
1 tsp lemon juice
250 gms/8.8ozs cooked mashed potato
1 cup warm water

For the icing:
75 gms/2.65oz butter
4.5 tbsp golden syrup
3 tsp ginger
1.5 tsp cinnamon
1.5 cup sifted icing sugar

Instructions

1. Preheat oven to 350°F/180°C.
2. Oil a set of muffin tins.
3. In a bowl, beat together the eggs, sugar, oil, lemon juice and golden syrup with egg beaters.
4. Sift all the dry ingredients together.
5. Add the wet to the dry ingredients and mix thoroughly.
6. Place the potato and water in a food processor and process until smooth.
7. Add to the main mixture.
8. Spoon into the muffin tins and bake 16-18 minutes until cooked through.
9. Remove gently from the muffin tins and cool on a rack.
10. Repeat until you have used up all the mixture.
11. Place all the icing ingredients into a saucepan and heat until melted.
12. When the muffins are cool and the icing has cooled a little, spread on top of the muffins.

Note: These will last longer than the usual day so freeze some of them and leave the rest out to be enjoyed.

Strands of My Life

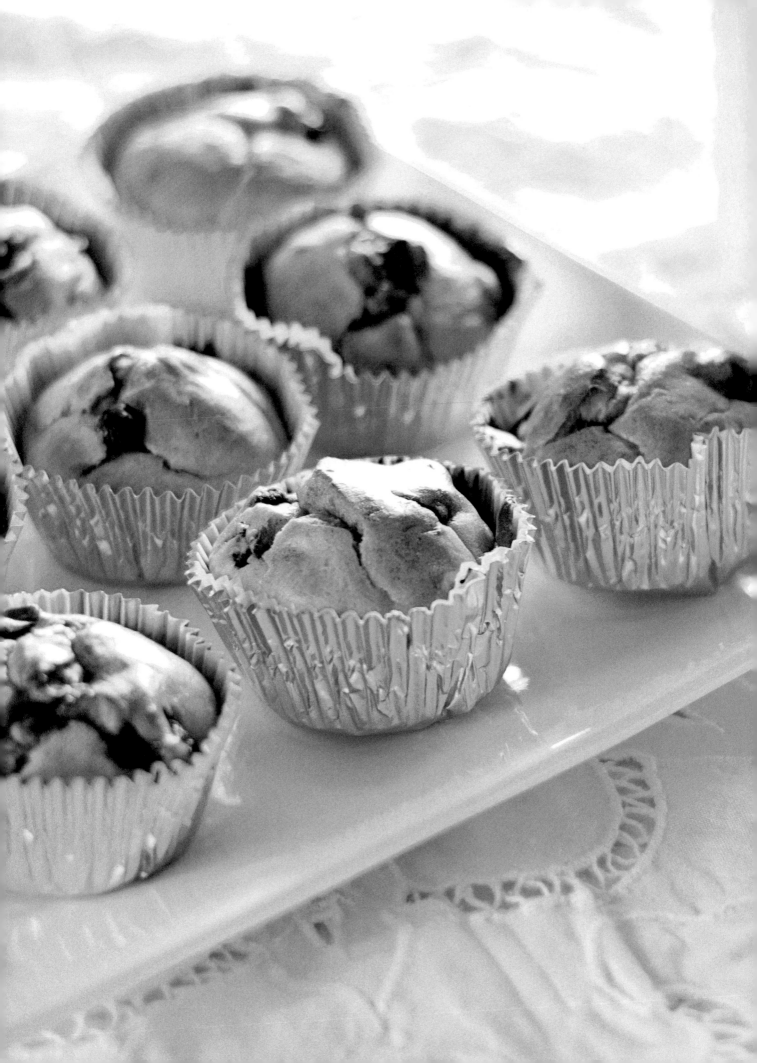

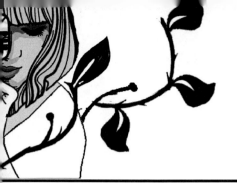

Peanut Butter & Banana Muffins

Ingredients

1 cup peanut butter
2 small bananas
2 large eggs
½ tsp baking powder
1 tsp vinegar
1 cup blueberries

Instructions

1. Preheat the oven to 180°C/350°F.
2. Place all the ingredients except the blueberries in a food processor and process until smooth.
3. Remove from the processor and fold in the blueberries.
4. Spoon into 12 muffin tins and bake for approx. 10 minutes.

Note: This recipe has no flour.

Makes 12 muffins

Strands of My Life

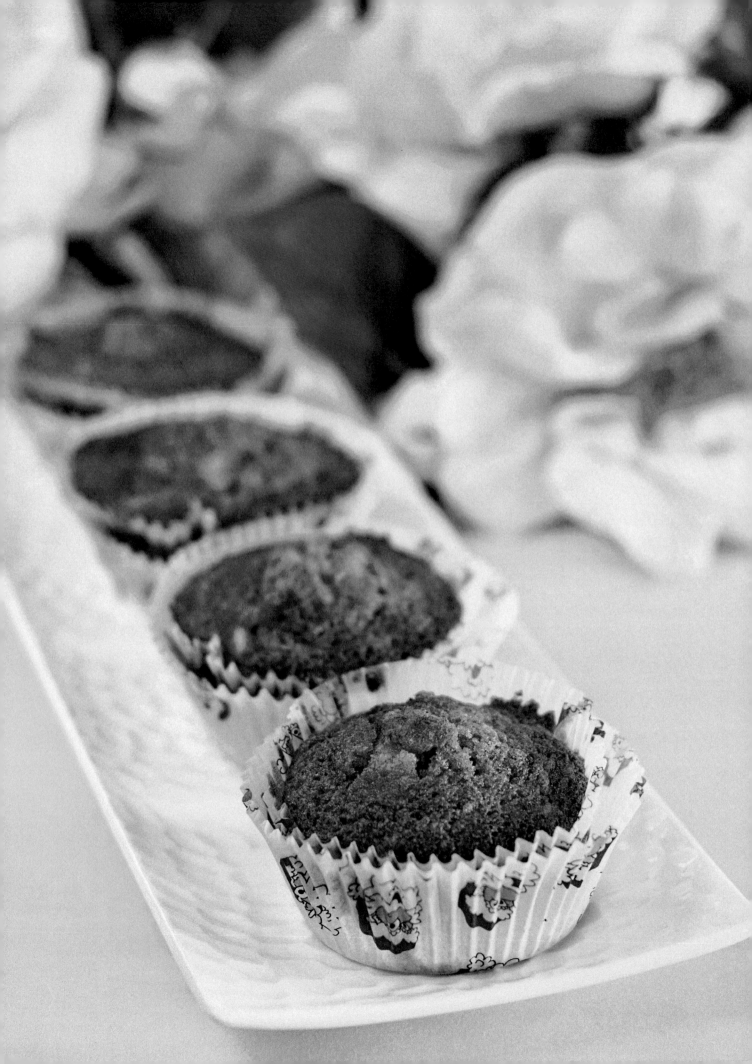

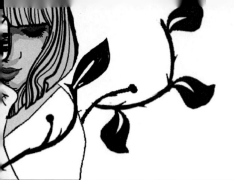

Carrot Cake Muffins

Ingredients

1.25 cups oil
1.5 cups white sugar
2.5 cups grated carrots
4 eggs
432gm/15oz can of unsweetened crushed pineapple
1.3 cups white rice flour
0.3 cup tapioca flour
0.3 cup potato starch
2 tsp cinnamon
1.5 tsp allspice
1 tsp ginger powder
1.5 tsp baking powder
2 tsp baking soda

Instructions

1. Preheat oven to 180°C/350°F.
2. Grease a muffin tin.
3. Grate the carrots.
4. Beat the sugar, oil and eggs together.
5. Add in the carrots and pineapple.
6. Sift all the dry ingredients together.
7. Blend the wet ingredients with the dry.
8. Spoon the mixture into the muffin tin.
9. Bake for 20 minutes or until a skewer comes out clean.
10. Turn out onto a cooling rack.

Note: These stay fresh for several days.

Makes 24 muffins

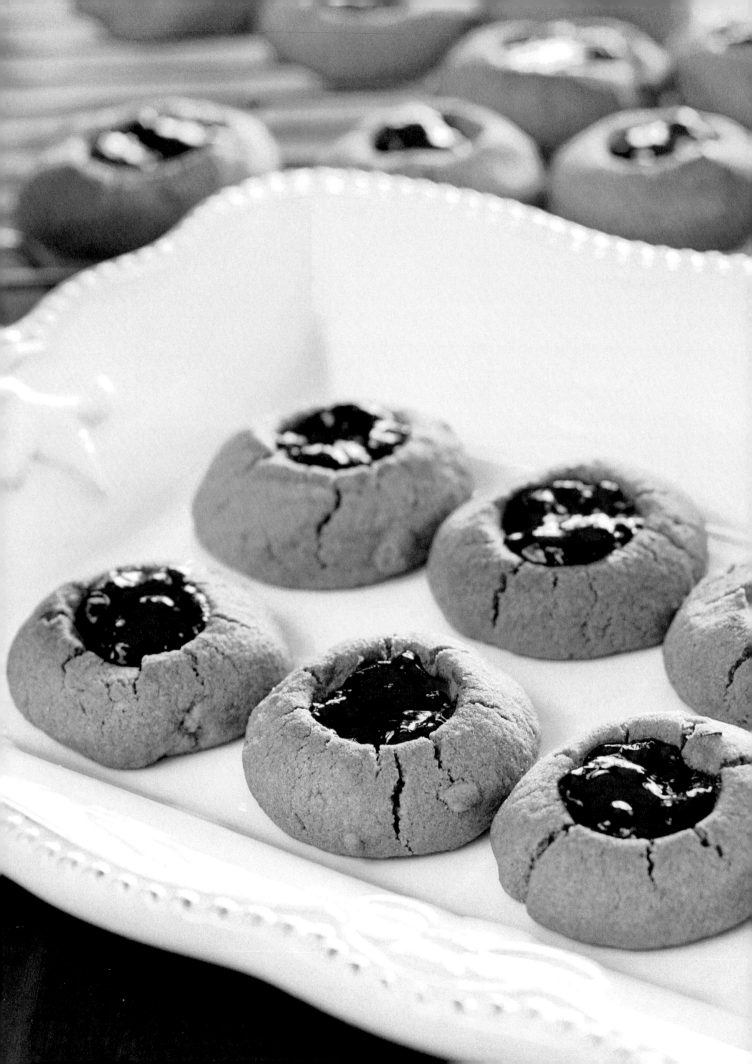

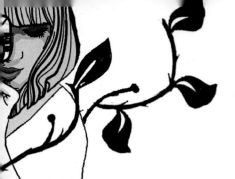

Thumbprint Cookies

Ingredients

2 cups white rice flour
½ cup potato starch
¼ cup tapioca flour
1/3 cup cocoa powder
pinch of salt
226gms/2 sticks butter
1 cup sugar
2 small eggs
2 tsp pure vanilla extract
sugarless blueberry jam

Instructions

1. Sift all the dry ingredients except the sugar into a bowl.
2. In a separate bowl, using egg beaters, beat softened butter and sugar until light in color and fluffy.
3. Add in egg and vanilla – continue beating until amalgamated well.
4. Add dry ingredients to the wet and mix well.
5. Roll dough into 1"/2.5cm balls and arrange on two oven trays lined with baking paper.
6. Press a hollow into a centre of each cookie using the end of a wooden spoon.
7. Place in the freezer for about 30 minutes.
8. Heat oven to 180°C/350°F.
9. Bake for 7 minutes then take the cookies out and press the hollow into the centre of each cookie again with the end of a wooden spoon.
10. Then bake for 5-7 more minutes.
11. Let cookies cool completely.
12. Place a small amount of jam into the hollow of each cookie.

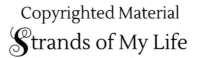
Strands of My Life

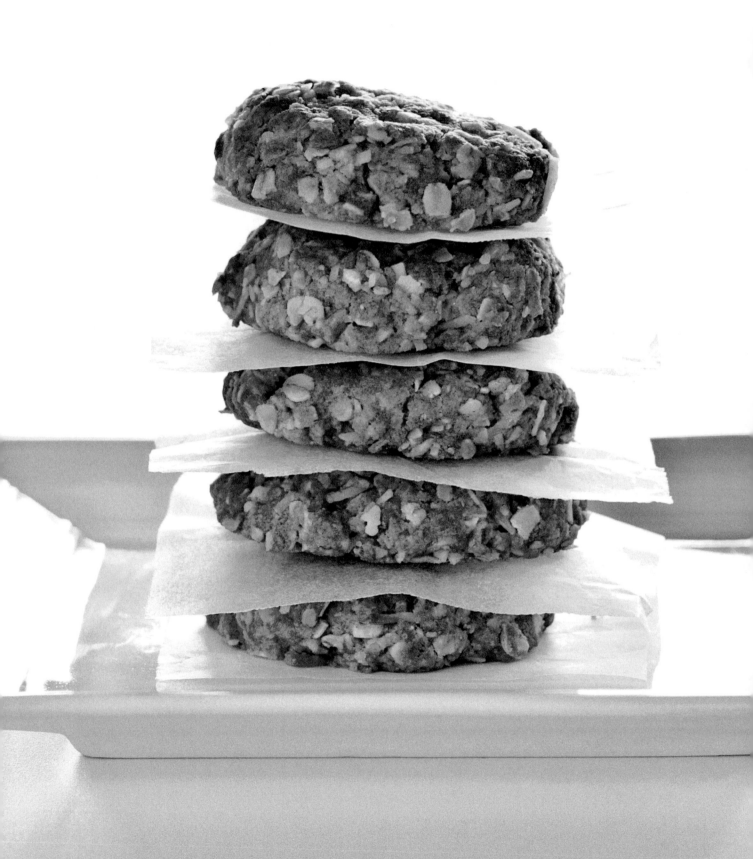

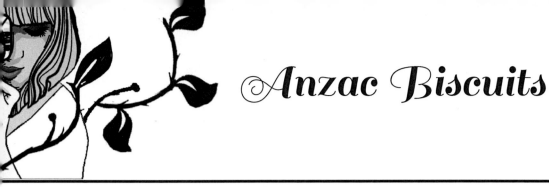

Anzac Biscuits

Ingredients

1 cup rolled oats
½ cup of white rice flour
¼ cup tapioca flour
¼ cup potato starch
1/3 cup cane sugar
¾ cup shredded coconut
2 tbsp golden syrup
125g/4oz butter
½ tsp baking soda
1 tbsp hot water

Instructions

1. Preheat the oven to 160°F/325°F.
2. Melt the butter with the golden syrup on the stove.
3. Mix the baking soda with the water to dissolve it.
4. Add to the butter mixture. It will froth up.
5. Combine the rest of the ingredients.
6. Mix the dry ingredients with the wet.
7. Line a baking tray with baking paper.
8. Place spoonfuls of the mixture on the tray and flatten slightly.
9. Bake for 10 minutes.
10. Remove and cool a little before moving to a cooling tray.

Strands of My Life

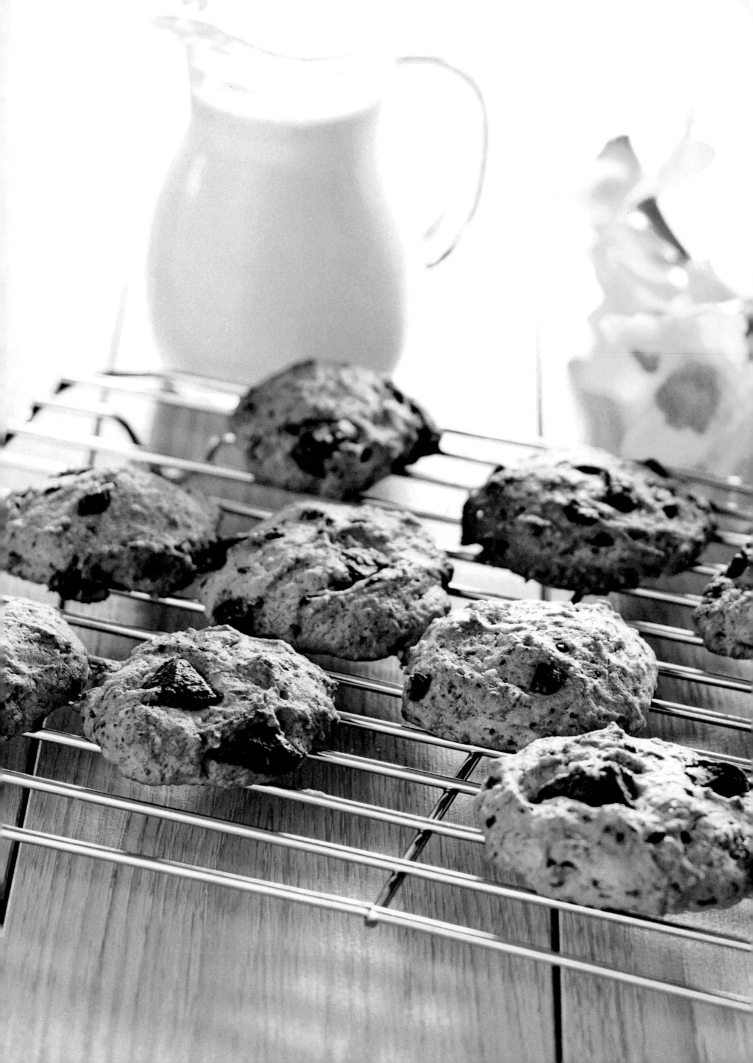

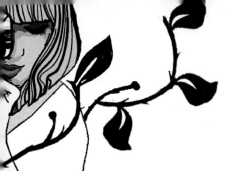

Chocolate Chip Cookies

Ingredients

65gms/2.3oz unsalted butter
1 large egg
½ tsp vanilla extract
½ cup white rice flour
½ cup brown rice flour
¼ cup tapioca flour
¼ cup potato starch
½ tsp baking soda
Pinch of salt
1 tsp cinnamon
1 cup dark chocolate, broken up

Instructions

1. Heat oven to 180°C/350°F.
2. Cream together the butter and sugar until light and fluffy.
3. Add the egg and beat again until well incorporated and the mixture becomes thick.
4. Add the vanilla and mix in. Sift all the dry ingredients together.
5. Mix the wet ingredients with the dry.
6. Add the chocolate and fold in.
7. Chill the mixture in the fridge for ½ an hour.
8. Line a baking tray with baking paper.
9. Roll the mixture into balls about the size of a ping pong ball and place on the tray. Flatten them a little.
10. Bake for 12 minutes.

Note: 4-5 squares of dark chocolate are low Fodmap

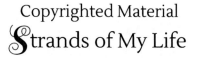

Strands of My Life

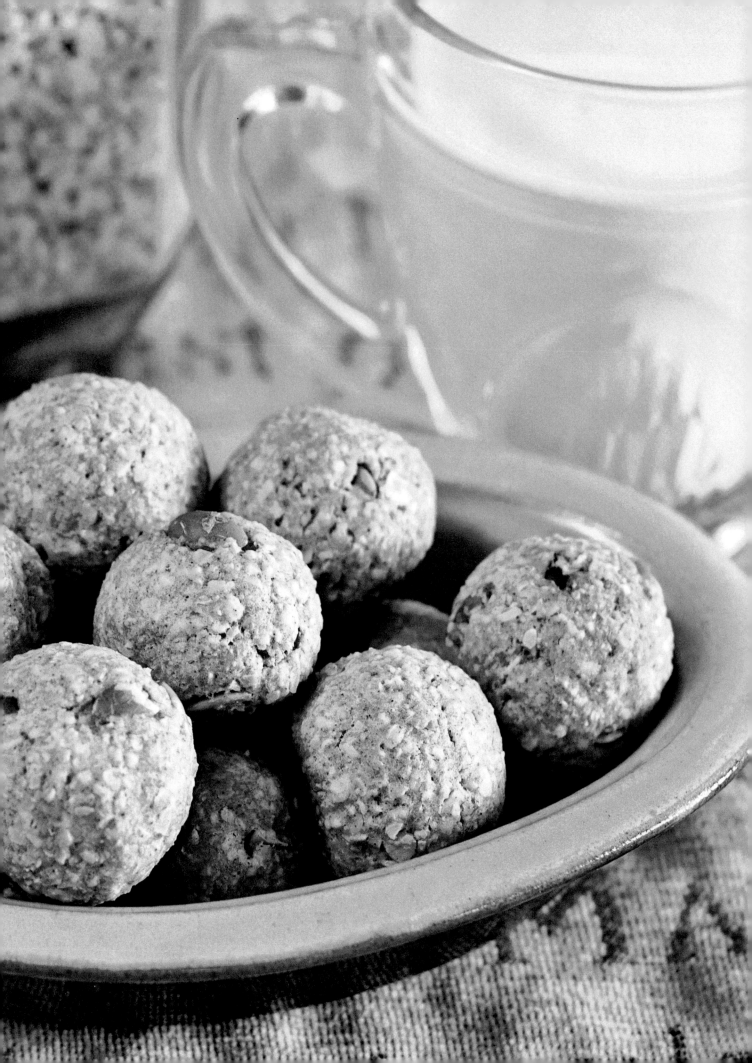

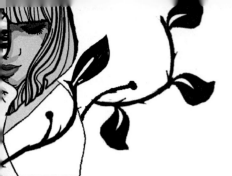

Banana Oat Truffles

Ingredients

2 cups instant oats
1 tbsp peanut butter
¼ cup tapioca flour
1 tbsp raw sugar
1 tbsp maple syrup
1/2 tsp cardamon
1/2 tsp ginger powder
1/2 tsp cinnamon
Pinch of salt
Pinch of chilli powder
½ cup of pumpkin seeds or chocolate chips

Instructions

1. Heat oven to 180°C/350°F.
2. Process the banana and peanut butter until well mixed.
3. Add all the dry ingredients and process again.
4. Rub a little oil onto your hands and roll the mixture into small balls.
5. Position them on an oven tray lined with baking paper.
6. Place in the oven and bake for 8 minutes.
7. Remove and eat warm or cool first. They are also great with some lactose-free Greek yoghurt.

NB: The bananas will vary in size so you may need to add a little more tapioca flour if they are too wet.

Makes 24 small balls

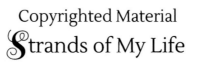

Strands of My Life

INDEX

Savoury Snacks

Sweet Snacks

Strands of
My Life
Combatting IBS with a Low Fodmap Diet

For more information on Suzanne Perazzini and her recipes, visit her food blog: www.strandsofmylife.com

If you would like to join her low Fodmap diet program, read about it on this page:
www.strandsofmylife.com/coachingprogram

OR

Go directly to this page to fill in the application form:
www.strandsofmylife.com/inspiredlife

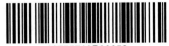

Made in the USA
San Bernardino, CA
10 March 2015